RESEARCH REPORT

District of Columbia Community Health Needs Assessment

Anita Chandra • *Janice C. Blanchard* • *Teague Ruder*

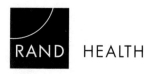

RAND HEALTH

The research described in this report was sponsored by the DC Healthy Communities Collaborative, and was conducted in RAND Health, a division of the RAND Corporation.

Library of Congress Cataloging-in-Publication Data

Chandra, Anita, author.
  District of Columbia community health needs assessment / Anita Chandra, Janice C. Blanchard, Teague Ruder.
    p. ; cm.
  Includes bibliographical references.
  ISBN 978-0-8330-8053-0 (pbk. : alk. paper)
  I. Blanchard, Janice C., author. II. Ruder, Teague, author. III. Rand Corporation, issuing body. IV. District of Columbia Healthy Communities Collaborative. V. Title.
  [DNLM: 1. Health Services Needs and Demand—District of Columbia—Statistics. 2. Health Behaviors—District of Columbia—Statistics. 3. Health Care Rationing—District of Columbia—Statistics. 4. Health Status—District of Columbia—Statistics. 5. Socioeconomic Factors—District of Columbia—Statistics. W 16]

  RA409
  614.4'2—dc23
                                                                    2013021781

The RAND Corporation is a nonprofit institution that helps improve policy and decisionmaking through research and analysis. RAND's publications do not necessarily reflect the opinions of its research clients and sponsors.

RAND® is a registered trademark.

Published 2013 by the RAND Corporation
1776 Main Street, P.O. Box 2138, Santa Monica, CA 90407-2138
1200 South Hayes Street, Arlington, VA 22202-5050
4570 Fifth Avenue, Suite 600, Pittsburgh, PA 15213-2665
RAND URL: http://www.rand.org/
To order RAND documents or to obtain additional information, contact
Distribution Services: Telephone: (310) 451-7002;
Fax: (310) 451-6915; Email: order@rand.org

Preface

This report summarizes a community health needs assessment (CHNA) for the District of Columbia (D.C.) developed for the DC Healthy Communities Collaborative (DCHCC), a network of four hospitals (Children's National Medical Center, Howard University Hospital, Providence Hospital, and Sibley Memorial Hospital) and two federally qualified health centers (FQHCs) (Community of Hope and Unity). The report documents trends in health needs and health service use among District children and adults, with particular attention paid to differences by age, race/ethnicity, ward, and hospital, where relevant. The findings should be of interest to a range of District stakeholders invested in improving health and health care in the city. The report may also be of interest to health services researchers or health care planners interested in conducting a community health needs assessment to drive local health decisionmaking.

This study was conducted in RAND Health. For more information about RAND Health, please visit www.rand.org/health or contact Jeffrey Wasserman, Vice President and Director of RAND Health, at Jeffrey@rand.org. For more information about this study, please contact the principal investigator, Anita Chandra, at Chandra@rand.org.

Contents

Figures

Tables

Summary

The DCHCC represents a unique collaboration among four D.C.-area hospitals (Children's National Medical Center, Howard University Hospital, Providence Hospital, and Sibley Memorial Hospital) and two FQHCs (Community of Hope and Unity). In spring 2013, an additional community health center—Bread for the City—joined the DCHCC membership. In response to its community commitment, current economic challenges, and new federal guidelines, DCHCC set forth to conduct a CHNA that summarizes and evaluates community health needs with attention to health status, health service needs, and the input of community stakeholders. CHNAs are increasingly used to lay a factual foundation for community health decisionmaking. The CHNA described in this report is intended to guide DCHCC's decisions about where and how to allocate resources and implement appropriate health interventions for the population served by the hospitals and FQHCs within DCHCC. It includes analysis of existing demographic, health status, and hospital service use data from the DC Health Matters (DCHM) portal,[1] supplemented by hospital and emergency department (ED) discharge data. We complement our analysis of these quantitative data with an analysis of current stakeholder perspectives regarding health need, as well as health policy and investment priorities. The key objectives of this written CHNA are as follows:

1. Describe the sociodemographics and health status of the population served by DCHCC with attention to differences by age, gender, race/ethnicity, and ward.
2. Examine inpatient and ED hospitalization rates to better understand patterns of health care use among residents of the local area with attention to differences by zip code, health care facility, and age, where relevant.
3. Describe the perspectives of community stakeholders with attention to barriers and facilitators to health service use and recommendations for health program and policy improvement.

Sociodemographic Trends

In 2011, the D.C. population totaled 617,996. Approximately 50 percent of the District's residents are black, 35 percent are white, 10 percent are Hispanic, and 4 percent are Asian. Overall, the proportion of District residents that is black decreased from 2000 to 2011 (from 59.5

---

[1] See http://www.dchealthmatters.org.

percent to 49.5 percent), while the proportion that is Hispanic grew slightly (from 7.9 percent to 9.5 percent), the proportion that is Asian grew from 2.6 percent to 3.6 percent, and the proportion that is white grew from 27.7 percent to 35.3 percent. Fifteen percent of District residents report speaking a language other than English at home.

Roughly 15 percent of the District's families live below the federal poverty level (FPL). The percentage of families who live in extreme poverty (or 185 percent of FPL) decreased from 2000 to 2011. Further, the percentage of residents who are college graduates sharply increased in the last decade (from 39 percent to 53 percent). The District population has become slightly younger, with the greatest growth (18.3 percent) among 18–39 year olds, but with a decrease of almost 8 percent in the population under 18 years old.

Health Needs and Risk Behaviors

We principally used the Behavior Risk Factor Surveillance System (BRFSS) survey and Youth Risk Behavior Survey (YRBS) to explore health needs and risk behaviors in the District. Where relevant, we also used data from the D.C. Department of Health, the National Center for Health Statistics, the Substance Abuse and Mental Health Services Administration (SAMHSA), and other local studies. Our findings focus on the areas of (1) general health quality and the use of preventive services, (2) nutrition and obesity, (3) chronic disease, (4) reproductive and sexual health, (5) mental health and substance use, (5) oral health, and (6) injuries.

General Health and the Use of Preventive Services

Insurance Status. As reported in previous health needs assessments, the District boasts a significantly smaller percentage of residents who are uninsured (7.7 percent) compared with the general U.S. population (18 percent). The number of children without insurance is also low relative to the U.S. population (7.5 percent of children nationally are uninsured as of 2011). According to the 2007 National Survey of Children's Health (the most recent survey wave available), approximately 3.5 percent of District children were uninsured. In 2009, the D.C. Department of Healthcare Finance estimated that approximately 60 percent of children ages 0–21 were publically insured.

Self-Reported Health. Only 3 percent of District residents (compared to 18 percent of U.S. residents) report only fair or poor health. In addition, fewer District residents on average note days of impairment in the past month due to poor physical health compared to the U.S. average (3.4 days versus 3.9 days). These impairment days are greatest among those 40 years of age or older.

Use of Preventive Health Services. The use of preventive health services is better in the District than nationwide (75 percent in the District had a routine checkup, compared to 67 percent in the United States). While these trends are generally positive, the percentage of older residents who have ever received a pneumococcal vaccine is less than the U.S. rate overall (63 percent in the District compared to 69 percent nationally), suggesting a possible point of health intervention. There are regional (by ward) differences in these outcomes.

Barriers to Care. Residents of some wards reported greater difficulty seeing a provider in the prior year due to cost. More 18–39 (11.2 percent) and 40–64 (11.6 percent) year olds missed care due to cost compared to those aged 65 years and older (5.7 percent).

Nutrition and Obesity

Obesity and Overweight. Black residents have a significantly higher rate of overweight and obesity as compared to white residents (66 percent black versus 40 percent white). Overweight and obesity is higher among those 40 years and older (62 percent) compared to those 18–39 years old (43 percent). Obesity is more prevalent in Wards 7 and 8 (21 percent and 32 percent, respectively), while general overweight is more prevalent in Wards 4 and 5 as compared to other wards (36 percent and 37 percent, respectively).

Exercise. Overall, District residents are more likely to report exercise in the prior month compared to the national average (80 percent in the District compared to 74 percent in the United States). However, self-reported rates of getting enough exercise are lowest among older adults in the District (70 percent of those 65 years and older compared to 86 percent of those 18–39 years old). District children between the ages of 6 and 17 were less likely to engage in physical activity (defined as 20 minutes or more of activity causing them to sweat) within the prior week compared to children in this age range nationally. Seventeen percent of District children between the ages of 4 and 17 reported no physical activity within the prior week as compared to 10.3 percent of children nationwide. Differences in these health behaviors across wards were also observed.

Chronic Disease and Disability

General Trends in Chronic Disease. Reported percentages of District residents with coronary heart disease, arthritis, and chronic obstructive pulmonary disorder (COPD) are lower than nationwide rates, but rates of asthma are higher (16 percent in the District compared to 14 percent in the United States). However, racial disparities were observed, with blacks having higher rates of heart disease, arthritis, COPD, and asthma. Ward differences were observed in the rates of most chronic diseases, particularly cardiovascular disease, asthma, diabetes, and emotional health limitations.

Cancer. In terms of the most recent 2009 data, the age-adjusted incidence of prostate and pancreatic cancers was higher in the District than the U.S. average. Lung and skin cancer incidence was lower in the District than in the nation. The incidence of pediatric cancer (all cancers among those younger than 20) is comparable to incidence nationwide. Blacks have considerably higher rates of cancer than whites in the District, as well as compared to overall rates nationwide.

Reproductive and Sexual Health

Reproductive Health. There were 9,156 births in the District in 2010, including 1,458 to mothers of Hispanic ethnicity (all races) and 4,940 to black mothers. Overall, the percentage of preterm births (prior to 37 weeks gestation) in the District declined from 16.0 percent of all births in 2006 to 13.6 percent of all births in 2010 (Martin et al., 2012). Infant mortality in 2010 was at its lowest rate in a decade, having declined from 10.6 per 1,000 live births in 2001 to 8.0 per 1,000 live births in 2010.

Sexual Health. The number of newly diagnosed human immunodeficiency virus (HIV) (including AIDS) cases has also declined in the past five years, as have deaths from HIV (including AIDS); the majority of new cases were among blacks. District residents report higher rates of HIV testing as compared to the rest of the country, and those rates are highest among those 18–39 years old. D.C. continues to report high rates of gonorrhea and chlamydia as compared to the rest of the country, with rates particularly high in Wards 7 and 8. Youth ages 15–19 have also accounted for an increase in the proportion of chlamydia and gonorrhea cases in the city over the past five years.

Mental Health and Substance Use

Mental Health. According to data from the 2010 and 2011 National Surveys of Drug Use and Health, 22.6 percent of District adults over the age of 18 reported any mental illness as compared to 19.8 percent of adults nationwide. Diagnosis of depressive disorder among adults also appears to be comparable to U.S. reports, although fewer people in the District report having the necessary social or emotional support (asked in the survey as "do you feel you have enough social or emotional support?" [45 percent in the District compared to 51 percent nationally]). Diagnosis of depressive disorder was more common among those 40–64 years old than among other age groups. More white adult residents than black residents report being diagnosed with depressive disorder (18 percent versus 15.4 percent). District youth have lower rates of feelings of sadness as compared to the rest of the country, with 23 percent of District high school students reporting feeling sad or hopeless for at least two weeks in the past 30 days compared to 28 percent of youth nationally.

Mental Health Service Use. According to a 2010 report about behavioral health care in the District, there is significant unmet need particularly for persons with mental illness and Medicaid managed care, DC Alliance, or those who lack insurance. Approximately 60 percent of adults and 72 percent of adolescents enrolled in Medicaid managed care plans were estimated to have an unmet need for depression care (Gresenz, 2010).

Smoking and Substance Abuse. Smoking is less common in the District compared to the United States overall. However, binge drinking and heavy drinking is more common, with a rate of 25 percent in the District for binge drinking compared to 18 percent in the United States and a rate of 10 percent for heavy drinking in the District compared to 6 percent in the United States). By age group, more 18–39-year-olds report binge and heavy drinking (39 percent binge; 13 percent heavy) and more 40–64-year-olds report being current smokers than other age groups (23 percent versus 11 percent of those 65 years and older and 21 percent for 18–39-year-olds). As with mental health diagnoses, there are also racial differences in substance use. More white residents than black residents report frequent engagement in binge (32 percent white versus 18 percent black) and heavy drinking (12 percent white versus 7 percent black). The District has higher rates of illicit drug use for all people ages 12 and above as compared to the United States nationwide, with 13.5 percent of District residents reporting any illicit drug use in the past 30 days as compared to 8.8 percent of residents nationwide.

Oral Health

More residents in the District have had a tooth removed due to decay (48 percent in the District compared to 45 percent in the United States); however, more residents also report having their teeth cleaned as compared to the overall U.S. rate (73 percent in the District versus 69 percent in the United States). In the District, rates of any dental visit, as well as preventive care dental visits, specifically among children covered by Medicaid, are low but comparable to the national average. The rate of having any teeth removed increases with age, with nearly 70 percent of those 65 years or older reporting that experience.

Injuries

General Injury Prevention. District residents engage in injury prevention behaviors similar to the rest of the country; however, black residents report a lower rate of seatbelt use (85 percent) as compared to white residents (89 percent). White residents are more likely to report falls than black residents (17 percent white versus 14 percent black), but there is no difference in falls by age.

Youth Violence. There was no difference between the United States overall and the District in terms of carrying weapons on school property, and fewer District youth reported being bullied at school (10 percent) compared to the U.S. report of 20 percent. On the other hand, more high school youth in the District reported physical abuse in intimate relationships (e.g., boyfriend/girlfriend) (15 percent versus 9 percent).

Violent Crime. The District has a higher violent crime rate as compared to the rest of the country, with 1,202.1 violent crimes per 100,000 population as compared to a national rate of 386.3 per 100,000 in 2011. The murder rate was also higher, with 17.5 murders per 100,000 in 2011 as compared to a rate of 4.7 per 100,000 nationwide. However, the District has observed a downward trend in the number of homicides, reaching a 20-year low of 78 total homicides in 2012 compared to 243 homicides in 2003 and 454 in 1993.

Health Service Use

Access to and Use of Preventive Services

The uninsurance rate is quite low in the District (7.7 percent) compared to the national uninsurance rate (16 percent). Sixty percent of those without insurance cited no regular source of care compared to only 15 percent of those with insurance. Fewer residents with insurance missed care due to cost. Cancer screenings (e.g., mammograms, pap smears, colonoscopies, prostate-specific antigen [PSA] tests) are more common among those with insurance than those without insurance.

Inpatient and Emergency Department Discharges

General Rates. From 2006 to 2011, overall inpatient discharge rates for D.C. residents remained fairly steady. However, when examined by age, rates among those 65 years and older fell from 299 to 269 per 1,000. For ED discharges, rates were also steady across age groups generally. However, discharge rates were steady among those 0–17 years old through 2009 and then increased substantially in 2010 and 2011.

Discharge Reasons. We examined the top reasons across all hospitals for inpatient and ED discharges. The top reasons for inpatient discharges are diseases of the heart, complications related to injury and poisoning, and pregnancy. For ED discharges, respiratory infections and contusions were frequently cited (the second and third most reported, respectively), though conditions without a clear diagnosis were the most common.

Ambulatory Care Sensitive Inpatient and ED Discharges

We use 2000–2011 DC Hospital Association (DCHA) data to describe trends in hospitalizations that are sensitive to the availability and effectiveness of outpatient services, such as primary and specialty care. These are referred to as ambulatory care sensitive (ACS) hospitalizations and are used as a proxy for the availability and use of primary and preventive health services. Often, rates of ACS hospitalizations are used to determine where need is high in a community, yet health service availability is low or health service use is inappropriate.

ACS Rates. Like overall inpatient and ED discharges, ACS inpatient discharges have sharply declined among those 65 years and older but have held steady across all other age groups. ACS ED discharges are greatest among those 0–17 years old, with a sharp increase in 2010 and 2011. This increase appears to have been driven predominantly by ED discharges in Ward 8, followed by Ward 7.

Asthma. For inpatient and ED discharges, asthma rates among those 0–17 years old experienced some decline in 2004 but have sharply increased since that point.

Diabetes. Diabetes is also a key condition for ACS calculations, particularly inpatient discharges. Overall, inpatient discharges related to diabetes have declined among the older age groups (40 years and older) and have held steady among younger age groups. By ward, there is a lot of "noise" in the inpatient discharges, particularly in Wards 7 and 8, among 0–17-year-olds, with sharp increases and decreases since 2006.

Sepsis and Cellulitis. Sepsis-related discharges are still high among those 65 years and older and are most common among those in Ward 5. The rate of cellulitis is also fairly high and generally steady among all age groups, with some increase since 2008 among those 0–17 years old.

Other Trends. One of the most notable trends over the last few years is a sharp decline in heart disease–related discharges, particularly those related to coronary atherosclerosis. A key trend in ED discharges in the past few years is in the area of "stress-related discharges," namely headaches, migraines, and back pain. Discharges related to these problems have all increased. For example, the rate of ED discharges due to back pain has sharply increased, especially among those 40–64 years old and is greatest in this age group among those in Wards 5, 6, and 7.

Visits to Federally Qualified Health Centers

Unity Health Care, Community of Hope, La Clinica del Pueblo, and Mary's Center are the four District grantees designated as FQHCs and captured in the national Uniform Data System (UDS) as of the time of this study. In 2011, there were a total of 122,891 patients served by these clinics, with 45 percent being male patients and 55 percent being female patients.

Stakeholder Perspectives

For this assessment, we also convened four focus groups with community stakeholders (e.g., leaders from community-based organizations, health and social service agencies, and faith-based groups) to discuss community health issues and recommendations for improvement. Our findings from these focus groups largely confirmed findings from our survey and hospital discharge data analysis. We identified nine common themes that emerged in our focus group discussions: (1) behavioral health, (2) obesity and nutrition, (3) preventive health services, (4) specialty services, (5) eldercare and end-of-life services, (6) disability services, (7) information technology, (8) case management, and (9) social determinants/social services.

Behavioral Health. Behavioral health services are limited for persons with Medicaid and persons for whom English is not their primary language. In particular, there are limited transitional services available to persons with behavioral health needs, especially among non-English speaking populations. More services are needed to help support community-based independent living for persons with behavioral health needs.

Obesity and Nutrition. There are few programs targeting obesity and promoting healthy eating. In particular, more programs should be developed that focus on the entire family.

Preventive Health Services. Focus group participants felt that hospitals in the District tended to focus on acute treatment services rather than preventive health care services. Hospitals should work with social service agencies to promote more programs that support healthy behaviors.

Specialty Services. There is a particular need for specialty services, such as pain management services and oncology services. The shortage of specialty services is greatest in Wards 7 and 8. Participants recommended provider practice incentives (such as loan repayment) and partnerships between hospitals and community-based health organizations to provide needed specialty services in areas where there are shortages.

Eldercare and End-of-Life Services. District residents who are primary caregivers for elderly family members have little support to help them provide effective home-based care. Case management efforts should focus on supporting eldercare. In addition, residents are often not aware of hospice and end-of-life services available in the community.

Disability Services. There are limited services available to support persons with disabilities in the city. Furthermore, health care providers are often ill equipped to treat this population due to a lack of medical education in this area. An expansion in the number of health and social service programs for persons with disabilities is needed.

Information Technology. There is little linkage of information systems across health care settings, often leading to duplicative services. More investment in a regional health information system is needed to help address this problem.

Case Management. There is little linkage of case management across hospitals to provide continuity of care for residents who may use services at multiple sites. There is also little linkage of hospitals to medical homes at discharge. There is a need for more-intensive patient navigation services to help residents make the greatest use of health services in the city.

Social Determinants/Social Services. A number of social determinants influence health care status in the city, including poverty, cultural differences, language, housing, and literacy. For hospitals and health care organizations to be most effective, providers must develop a greater awareness of these social determinants and their impact on the health of District residents. Programs that target these social determinants are needed, including greater cultural competency training and health interventions more appropriately tailored to the languages and literacy levels of District residents.

Conclusion

The CHNA revealed six priority areas: asthma, obesity, mental health, sexual health, stress related disorders (e.g., headache, back pain), and general access to health services. We determined priority areas by using a combination of quantitative (administrative, survey) and qualitative (focus group) data analysis, as well as considering broader national health priority areas, paying particular attention to issues that have persisted over the last decade or experienced a recent increase or spike in the District. Despite high insurance rates, health care services are not evenly distributed by ward, creating significant challenges to access. In particular, specialty services such as oncology and pain management services are lacking in Wards 7 and 8. There is a need for the expansion of these services, as well as greater care coordination between health and social services to help residents navigate the system and obtain needed services.

Acknowledgments

We would like to thank our project sponsor, the D.C. Healthy Communities Collaborative, for its support of this research. This includes Children's National Medical Center, Howard University Hospital, Providence Hospital, Sibley Memorial Hospital, Community of Hope, and Unity Health Care. In addition, we extend our appreciation to Chaya Merrill and Ruth Pollard for their leadership of this effort. We express gratitude to the community stakeholders who participated in our focus groups and Machelle Yingling from the D.C. Hospital Association for providing critical hospital data.

We appreciate the thoughtful reviews of Vivian Towe at RAND and Monika Goyal at Children's National Medical Center.

Abbreviations

ACS	ambulatory care sensitive
ACSY	American Community Survey
BMI	body mass index
BRFSS	Behavior Risk Factor Surveillance System
CDC	Centers for Disease Control and Prevention
CHIP	Children's Health Insurance Program
CHNA	Community Health Needs Assessment
CMS	Centers for Medicare and Medicaid Services
COPD	chronic obstructive pulmunary disorder
D.C.	District of Columbia
DCHA	DC Hospital Association
DCHCC	DC Healthy Communities Collaborative
DCHM	DC Health Matters
DOH	Department of Health
ED	emergency department
FPL	federal poverty level
FQHC	Federally Qualified Health Center
HIV	human immunodeficiency virus
HPSA	health professional shortage area
HRSA	Health Resources and Services Administration
IDU	injection drug use
KFF	Kaiser Family Foundation
MUA/MUP	medically underserved areas/populations
PSA	prostate specific antigen
RHIO	Regional Health Information Organization
SE	standard error
STI	sexually transmitted infection
UDS	Uniform Data System
YRBS	Youth Risk Behavior Survey

CHAPTER ONE

Introduction

The District of Columbia (D.C.) Healthy Communities Collaborative (DCHCC) represents a unique collaboration between four D.C.-area hospitals (Children's National Medical Center, Howard University Hospital, Providence Hospital, and Sibley Memorial Hospital) and two Federally Qualified Health Centers (FQHCs) (Community of Hope and Unity). In spring 2013, an additional community health center—Bread for the City—joined the DCHCC membership. In response to its community commitment, current economic challenges, and new federal guidelines, DCHCC set forth to conduct a Community Health Needs Assessment (CHNA) that summarizes and evaluates community health needs with attention to health status, health service needs, and the input of community stakeholders. The following report addresses the requirements for a CHNA as outlined in the Affordable Care Act of 2010 and as part of 501(c)(3) standards for nonprofit hospitals. The scope of this project also includes support for an innovative data-reporting website and tool that will engage many different stakeholders committed to improving health outcomes in the District of Columbia.

CHNAs are increasingly used to lay a factual foundation for community health decision-making. This CHNA is intended to guide DCHCC's decisions about where and how to allocate resources and implement appropriate health interventions for the population served by the hospitals and FQHCs within DCHCC (i.e., within their catchment area). CHNAs also integrate multiple data streams, thus augmenting the value of their recommendations and helping to prioritize where investments should be made based on both health need and service data.

The CHNA described in this report includes analysis of existing demographic, health status, and hospital service use data from the DC Health Matters (DCHM) portal, supplemented by hospital and emergency department (ED) discharge data. We also complement these quantitative data with an analysis of current stakeholder perspectives regarding health needs, as well as health policy and investment priorities. In this report, we define *community* as the populations served by local D.C. hospitals and community health centers, specifically those individuals residing within the District.

The key objectives of this CHNA are as follows:

1. Describe the sociodemographics and health status of the population served by DCHCC with attention to differences by age, gender, race/ethnicity, and ward.
2. Examine inpatient and ED hospitalization rates to better understand patterns of health care use among residents of the local area with attention to differences by zip code, health care facility, and age, where relevant.

3. Describe the perspectives of community stakeholders with attention to barriers and facilitators to health service use and recommendations for health program and policy improvement.
4. Develop an interactive, electronic web-based version of the CHNA that can be tailored to the specific needs of community stakeholders.

This report focuses on the first three objectives, with particular emphasis on health and health care determinants. We offer some context on the social determinants of health via discussion of our focus groups (Chapter Five), but this report focuses proportionately more attention on health needs, health service use patterns, and the reasons for those needs and patterns. Additional data on the metrics of community health and social determinants are provided in the DCHM. Table 1.1 profiles the data sources used in this report, including the Behavioral Risk Factor Surveillance System (BRFSS), the American Community Survey (ACSY), and data from the DC Hospital Association (DCHA) on inpatient and ED discharges. We supplement these data with information on key indicators from other sources, such as vital statistics and other community health reports.

Table 1.1
Key Data Sources

Data Source	Time Period	Description
ACSY; Decennial Census	2006–2011	We analyzed data from the 2000 and 2010 Decennial Censuses, as well as the 2006–2011 ACSY, to highlight changes in the sociodemographic composition of District residents over time.
BRFSS	2000–2011	We conducted analyses of BRFSS's self-reported data on health, preventive health use, mental health and substance use, nutrition and obesity, and injuries for District residents aged 18 and older. For ward differences, we relied on summary reports from the D.C. Department of Health based on the 2010 BRFSS. All other tables use the 2011 BRFSS, of which the study team conducted its own analyses. Items varied year-to-year in some cases, as noted in the tables where relevant. For analyses by location (D.C. versus the entire United States), age, and race/ethnicity, statistical testing was conducted. For ward analyses for which we did not have data, we do not report p-values.
Youth Risk Behavior Survey (YRBS)	2008–2011	We summarized YRBS data for high school (9th–12th grade) students using information from the Centers for Disease Control and Prevention (CDC). Where relevant, we provide trends, though with question wording changes, we primarily compare D.C. and U.S. rates in 2011.
DCHA	2000–2011	We analyzed inpatient and ED discharge data from DCHA. This includes all hospitals in the District, but does not include ED data from the United Medical Center. We supplemented DCHA data with ED data from Children's National Medical Center. Our analysis used the 2002 Ward boundaries for District of Columbia.
Focus groups with community organization leaders	2012	We conducted four focus groups with community organization leaders (from a range of health and social services, faith-based groups, and other community organizations). The focus groups used a semistructured protocol. Two focus groups on health care issues; two emphasized social determinants of health.

Chapter Two provides background information on the basic sociodemographic characteristics of District residents. Chapter Three describes information related to health and health risk behaviors. Chapter Four describes health care use patterns and Chapter Five summarizes perspectives from D.C. organization leaders. Chapter Six provides conclusions and brief recommendations.

Sociodemographic Characteristics and Trends in the District

This chapter briefly describes the demographic characteristics of District residents. The analyses are based on data from the 2000 and 2010 Decennial Censuses, as well as the annual ACSY through 2011.[1] Section 2.2 presents sociodemographic characteristics of District residents by ward and over time.

2.1 Geography of the District

The District is composed of 100 zip codes, and is divided into 8 wards corresponding to electoral districts (Figure 2.1). However, there are only 22 core residential ZIP codes; the rest are unique to office buildings, universities, military bases, or post office boxes. In this report, we present data by ward, using ward–to–ZIP code matching.

2.2 Sociodemographic Characteristics of District Residents

In 2011, the D.C. population totaled 617,996. Table 2.1 details the population's sociodemographic characteristics: 49.5 percent of the District's residents are black, 35 percent are white, 10 percent are Hispanic, and 4 percent are Asian. Overall, the proportion of District residents that is black decreased between 2000 and 2011 from 59.5 percent to 49.5 percent, while the proportion that is Hispanic grew slightly from 7.9 percent to 9.5 percent, the proportion that is Asian grew from 2.6 percent to 3.6 percent, and the proportion that is white grew from 27.7 percent to 35.3 percent. Table 2.2 presents characteristics across the eight District wards. In Wards 7 and 8, more than 10 times the number of residents live in poverty than in Ward 3 (23.3 percent and 32.0 percent, respectively). Wards 7 and 8 continue to comprise mostly black residents, while Ward 1 has a large Hispanic population. In addition, Ward 1 has the largest percentage of individuals who are foreign born (22.4 percent) and individuals who speak a language other than English at home (23.2 percent).

Overall, the District population has become slightly younger, with the greatest growth among 18–39-year-olds (18.3 percent from 2000 to 2011), but with a decrease of almost 8 percent in the population under 18 years old. Figure 2.2 demonstrates the age distribution of this population by ward, using analyses of aggregated ACSY data from 2006 to 2010. As shown

---

[1] The ACSY collects data annually between decennial censuses and allows for the sociodemographic characteristics of District residents to be summarized at the ward level.

**Figure 2.1
District Wards (2002)**

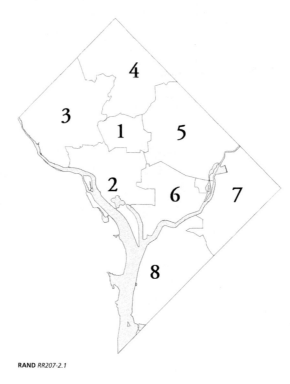

RAND *RR207-2.1*

in Figure 2.2, Wards 7 and 8 have the largest proportion of their population represented by 0–17-year-olds. Wards 4 and 5 have the largest proportion of their population represented by those older than 65 years.

**Figure 2.2
Age Distribution by Ward (2006–2010)**

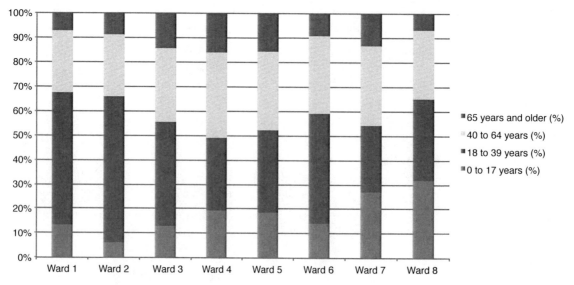

SOURCE: Aggregated ACSY data.
RAND *RR207-2.2*

Table 2.1
Sociodemographic Changes in the District (2000–2011)

Characteristic		2000	2011
Age	0–17 years (%)	20.0	**17.1**
	18–39 years (%)	38.6	**42.3**
	40–64 years (%)	29.2	29.4
	65 years and older (%)	12.3	**11.3**
Race and ethnicity	Black, non-Hispanic (%)	59.5	**49.5**
	White, non-Hispanic (%)	27.7	**35.3**
	Asian, non-Hispanic (%)	2.6	**3.6**
	Hispanic (%)	7.9	**9.5**
	Foreign born (%)	12.9	13.5
	Speak a language other than English at home (individuals aged 5 and older) (%)	16.8	**15.0**
Family income	Below poverty level (%)	16.7	15.4
	Below 1.85 times poverty level (%)*	29.6	**25.7**
	Median household income ($)	40,127.0	63,124.0
Education (adults aged 25 and older)	Less than high school (%)	22.2	**12.8**
	High school diploma or equivalent (%)	20.6	**17.7**
	Some college (%)	18.2	17.0
	College graduate (%)	39.1	**52.5**

SOURCE: U.S. Bureau of the Census, Decennial Census, 2000; American Community Survey, 2011.

NOTE: Bolded figures indicate statistically significant change from 2000 to 2011 (with 95 percent confidence).
*Often the threshold for federal aid programs, including food assistance.

Roughly 15 percent of the District's families live below the poverty line. Yet, the percentage of families who live in extreme poverty (or 185 percent of federal poverty level [FPL]) decreased from 2000 to 2011 (Table 2.1). The unemployment rate is highest in Ward 7 (19 percent) (Table 2.2).

Finally, the percentage of residents who are college graduates sharply increased in the last decade (from 39 to 53 percent). Ward 3 has the largest proportion of individuals who have a college degree (83 percent), while Ward 8 has the largest proportion with less than a high school education (20 percent).

Table 2.2
Sociodemographic Characteristics of District Residents by Ward (2006–2010)

Characteristic		Ward 1	Ward 2	Ward 3	Ward 4	Ward 5	Ward 6	Ward 7	Ward 8
Population	Total population	72,467	73,632	78,508	74,194	72,334	76,994	68,574	67,697
	Percentage of District population	12.4	12.6	13.4	12.7	12.4	13.2	11.7	11.6
Age	0–17 years (%)	13.5	6.0	12.9	19.3	18.5	14.2	27.0	31.9
	18–39 years (%)	54.1	60.0	42.4	29.7	33.7	44.8	27.4	33.3
	40–64 years (%)	25.1	25.3	30.2	34.9	32.1	31.6	32.3	28.1
	65 years and older (%)	7.2	8.8	14.5	16.0	15.7	9.3	13.3	6.7
Race and ethnicity	Black, non-Hispanic (%)	35.0	14.5	4.9	61.6	79.4	43.8	95.3	93.6
	White, non-Hispanic (%)	38.1	65.2	77.2	18.3	11.3	44.0	1.5	3.1
	Asian, non-Hispanic (%)	12.0	6.9	6.3	5.3	2.4	3.0	0.5	0.6
	Hispanic (%)	20.5	9.3	7.7	16.4	5.8	5.4	2.1	2.2
	Foreign born (%)	22.4	18.6	17.7	20.1	8.8	9.1	3.2	2.7
	Speak a language other than English at home (individuals aged 5 and older) (%)	23.2	20.7	20.4	22.0	8.6	11.6	3.9	3.8
Family income	Below poverty level (%)	13.0	4.5	2.1	7.0	14.5	14.8	23.3	32.0
	Below 1.85 times poverty level (%)	27.1	11.9	3.4	18.8	27.0	21.2	38.4	51.9
	Child poverty (%)*	23.0	18.0	3.1	7.6	29.0	31.0	40.0	48.0
	Unemployment (%)*	7.2	4.0	3.4	7.6	13.0	8.4	19.0	17.0
	Median household income ($)	64,973.0	76,870.0	97,257.0	58,668.0	47,402.0	78,449.0	36,828.0	30,653.0

Table 2.2—Continued

Characteristic		Ward 1	Ward 2	Ward 3	Ward 4	Ward 5	Ward 6	Ward 7	Ward 8
Education (adults aged 25 and older)	Less than high school (%)	17.5	7.6	3.1	16.5	17.8	11.4	17.3	20.3
	High school diploma or equivalent (%)	12.0	6.8	4.5	21.6	28.6	15.0	37.9	44.1
	Some college (%)	12.8	10.9	8.6	20.7	23.8	14.3	28.0	24.1
	College graduate (%)	57.7	74.7	83.8	41.2	29.7	59.3	16.8	11.6

SOURCE: U.S. Bureau of the Census, American Community Survey 2006–2010.
*Pooled data, 2005–2009.

CHAPTER THREE

Health and Health Risk Behaviors in the District

In this chapter, we use a number of data sources to present health indicators for District residents. We principally relied on BRFSS and YRBS data to document health status. The BRFSS and YRBS are key sources of health status data, which provide information about a wide range of health behaviors, including drug and alcohol use, smoking, nutrition, physical activity, and injury. In addition, we compiled information from existing reports published by the District of Columbia Department of Health (DOH) and the Centers for Disease Control and Prevention (CDC) to present statistics both for the city overall and by ward for other important health indicators, including rates of infant mortality, low birth weight, births to mothers under the age of 20, and human immunodeficiency virus (HIV) and sexually transmitted infection (STI) rates for District residents. In particular, we draw data from two recently published DOH reports: the *2010 Infant Mortality Rate for the District of Columbia* (DOH, 2012) and the *2011 Annual Report: HIV/AIDS, Hepatitis, STD, and TB Epidemiology in the District of Columbia* (DOH, 2011).

For adults, BRFSS provides good health status and chronic disease data. We offer ward comparisons for BRFSS information using 2010 data (DOH-generated data; 2010 BRFSS Annual Report; DOH, 2012), where relevant. In addition, we provide statistics on children generated using the YRBS data. In each section, we draw comparisons with the overall United States and assess differences by age, race/ethnicity, and ward, when applicable.

This analysis has two components of note. First, for BRFSS data, we only conducted significance testing when comparing District data to the United States as a whole and when making racial/ethnicity and age comparisons using District data. This is due to the fact that we had access to raw data files for analyses. When comparing wards, we did not benefit from this level of statistical analysis because raw data were not available; thus, we summarize the DOH (2012) report only. The ward differences from the DOH report are presented unadjusted (i.e., not controlled for age, race/ethnicity). For YRBS data, we were able to examine gender differences at $p<0.05$. In addition, for race/ethnicity comparisons, we only report differences between non-Hispanic, black, and white residents. The sample size for Hispanic residents is small, and thus it is difficult to conduct robust and reliable comparisons based on race/ethnicity for that category.

We begin with BRFSS adult data and include youth data from YRBS where appropriate. Sections are organized around the following health status core domains of interest:

- general health quality and the use of preventive services
- nutrition and obesity
- chronic disease

- reproductive and sexual health
- mental health and substance use
- oral health
- injuries.

We selected these domains based on prior CHNA groupings and the objectives of Healthy People 2020. For example, nutrition and weight status is a key area for improvement in Healthy People 2020 (e.g., increase the number of individuals at healthy weight, decrease the proportion of 12–19-year-olds considered obese to 16.5 percent). Under the domain of chronic disease, some key illnesses are diabetes, asthma, and cancer, all of which are addressed in this report.

In addition to the prevalence data, we provide some illustrative maps of assets and vulnerabilities related to each health domain of interest. For example, in the nutrition section, we include a figure that shows the distribution of food outlets. The scope of this report and its associated resources did not allow for robust analyses of these data (see Chandra et al., 2009, for example of health environment indices); thus we present these maps as illustrative tools with minimal interpretation and contextualization.

Finally, note that in the tables that show comparisons between the District and the United States, as well as comparisons by race/ethnicity and age, we list p-values and standard errors (SEs). The p-value is the probability that the difference between two groups is not due to chance. The SE is the standard deviation of those sample means over all possible samples (of a given size) drawn from the population.

3.1 General Health Quality and Access to Preventive Services Among District Residents

Table 3.1 summarizes key dimensions of self-reported health and the use of preventive services in the District and in the United States overall. Self-reported health status is one way to evaluate the population's overall health and has been found to be predictive of population mortality (McGee et al., 1999). Survey respondents indicated whether their overall health was excellent, very good, good, fair, or poor. Thirteen percent of District residents report fair or poor health versus 18 percent of U.S. residents. In addition, District residents note fewer days of impairment in the past month on average due to poor physical health (3.4 days versus 3.9 days). These impairment days are greatest among those 40 years old and above (Table 3.2). District residents also report fewer missed routine checkups and the lack of a personal health care provider. Younger adults in the District (those 64 years old and under) report more often missing care due to cost than older adults in the District. As in previous health needs assessments, the District boasts a significantly smaller percentage of residents who are uninsured[1] as compared to the general U.S. population. While these trends are positive, the percentage of older residents who have ever received a pneumococcal vaccine is less than the U.S. rate overall, suggesting a

---

[1]   Because BRFSS only asks a single question about insurance coverage (without listing potential sources of coverage by name, for example), it is unclear whether individuals in the alliance count themselves as insured or uninsured. BRFSS measures insurance at a particular point in time during the year rather than measuring insurance status for an entire year (as the Current Population Survey does).

Table 3.1
Adult Health Status and Preventive Service Use in D.C. Versus the United States

Variable	District of Columbia			United States			
	N	Mean or Percentage	SE	N	Mean or Percentage	SE	P-value
Days of poor mental health in the last 30 days	4,494	3.6	0.2	494,674	3.9	0.0	0.1903
Days of poor physical health in the last 30 days	4,475	3.4	0.2	492,260	3.9	0.0	0.0003
Missed care in the last 12 months because of cost	4,552	10.5%	0.8	503,102	17.0%	0.1	<.0.001
Self-rated health = Fair or Poor	4,522	13.7%	0.8	502,410	18.2%	0.1	<.0.001
No routine checkup in the past year	4,535	25.4%	1.0	497,817	33.1%	0.1	<.0.001
No personal health care provider	4,546	19.3%	1.0	502,806	22.0%	0.1	0.0090
Pneumococcal vaccine ever among adults 65 and older	1,261	63.3%	1.7	145,093	69.0%	0.2	0.0010
Flu shot or flu spray in the last year among adults 65 and older	1,342	56.7%	1.8	150,157	60.2%	0.2	0.0516
Uninsured	4,545	7.7%	0.7	502,756	18.3%	0.1	<.0.001

SOURCE: BRFSS, 2011.

NOTE: N = total BRFSS sample. P-values in bold indicate that the difference between the United States and the District is statistically significant for p<0.05.

possible point of health intervention. Please note that the sample size (n) provided in the tables denotes the number of individuals who responded to the question.

While BRFSS does not categorize individuals by type of insurance, the Kaiser Family Foundation (KFF) estimated that, as of 2010–2011, approximately 48 percent of District residents aged 0–64 years had employer-sponsored coverage, 7 percent had individually purchased private coverage, 10 percent were covered by Medicare, and 24 percent were covered by Medicaid (Kaiser Family Foundation, undated). The KFF rate of uninsurance in the District of 11 percent and the BRFSS rate of 7.7 percent are less than the corresponding rates of 16 percent (KFF) and 18 percent (BRFSS) uninsurance for the United States overall.

The number of children in the District without insurance is also low. According to the 2007 National Survey of Children's Health, approximately 3.5 percent of District children were uninsured. In 2009, the District of Columbia Department of Healthcare Finance estimated that approximately 60 percent of children ages 0–21 were publically insured. As of May 31, 2009, 85,793 children (ages 0–21) were covered by Medicaid and 1,944 children were covered by D.C. Alliance. All children covered by D.C. Alliance and nearly all children with Medicaid are covered by Medicaid managed care plans. In 2009, nearly 13,000 children were covered by Medicaid fee-for-service, mainly children with disabilities not enrolled in Health Services for Children with Special Needs (HSCSN) (personal communication with the Department of Health Care Finance cited in Chandra [2009]).

Table 3.3 describes differences in measures of health status by race/ethnicity, principally comparing white and black residents given the overall proportion in the District and the sample size for the BRFSS. While the overall rates were better in the District compared to the nation,

Table 3.2
D.C. Adult Health Status and Preventive Service by Age

Variable	18–39 Years			40–64 Years			65 Years and Older			P-value
	N	Mean or Percentage	SE	N	Mean or Percentage	SE	N	Mean or Percentage	SE	
Days of poor mental health in the last 30 days	879	3.76	0.35	2,118	3.85	0.25	1,421	2.53	0.27	0.0003
Days of poor physical health in the last 30 days	881	2.10	0.26	2,125	4.18	0.25	1,391	5.08	0.33	<.0001
Missed care in the last 12 months because of cost	888	11.2%	1.5	2,140	11.6%	1.0	1,442	5.7%	0.8	<.0001
Self-rated health = Fair or Poor	887	8.4%	1.3	2,143	8.7%	1.0	1,434	3.5%	0.6	<.0001
No routine checkup in the past year	886	29.1%	2.0	2,144	12.7%	1.1	1,435	6.8%	0.9	<.0001
No personal health care provider	882	31.5%	2.0	2,136	24.1%	1.3	1,435	11.0%	0.9	<.0001
Flu shot or flu spray in the last year among adults 65 and older	—	—	—	—	—	—	—	56.7%	1.8	—
Pneumococcal vaccine ever among adults 65 and older	—	—	—	—	—	—	—	63.3%	1.7	—
Have insurance	829	82.7%	1.9	2,027	88.5%	1.1	1,350	89.9%	1.0	<.0001

SOURCE: BRFSS, 2011.

NOTE: N = total BRFSS sample. P-values in bold indicate that the difference between at least two age categories is statistically significant for p<0.05.

there are significant racial/ethnic disparities. Black residents report more days of impairment due to both mental health issues (4.5 days versus 2.2 days) and physical health issues (4.4 days versus 2.0 days) than white residents. Black residents also reported poorer health, lower rates of pneumococcal or flu vaccination, and more missed care in the past 12 months due to cost than white residents. Accordingly, black residents were three times more likely to report having no insurance.

These health outcomes appeared different by ward, though statistical testing was not applied (Table 3.4). Using 2010 data (DOH, 2012), those residents in Wards 1 (27.0 percent) and 3 (29.3 percent) more frequently reported not having a routine checkup in the past year than in other wards. About 20 percent of individuals in Ward 5 reported not having a personal health care provider. About 13 percent of residents in Ward 7 and 16 percent of residents in Ward 8 reported missing care in the last 12 months because of cost.

Table 3.3
D.C. Adult Health Status and the Use of Preventive Services by Race/Ethnicity

Variable	White, Non-Hispanic			Black, Non-Hispanic			
	N	Mean or Percentage	SE	N	Mean or Percentage	SE	P-value
Days of poor mental health in the last 30 days	1,982	2.2	0.1	1,994	4.5	0.3	<.0001
Days of poor physical health in the last 30 days	1,980	2.0	0.2	1,980	4.4	0.3	<.0001
Missed care in the last 12 months because of cost	1,997	5.1%	0.8	2,029	14.8%	1.4	<.0001
Self-rated health = Fair or Poor	1,992	5.3%	0.7	2,005	20.7%	1.3	<.0001
Flu shot or flu spray in the last year among adults 65 and older	602	69.6%	2.1	651	48.4%	2.6	<.0001
No routine checkup in the past year	1,988	34.1%	1.6	2,024	17.3%	1.4	<.0001
No personal health care provider	1,995	19.7%	1.5	2,027	17.0%	1.6	0.0241
Pneumococcal vaccine ever among adults 65 and older	559	72.6%	2.2	618	57.6%	2.6	<.0001
Uninsured	1,995	3.4%	0.6	2,023	10.6%	1.2	<.0001

SOURCE: BRFSS, 2011.
NOTE: P-values in bold indicate that the difference between the black and white residents is statistically significant for p<0.05.

3.2 Nutrition and Obesity

We also examined rates of obesity, overweight, and general engagement in preventive activities for healthy lifestyles, including routine exercise and healthy eating. Table 3.5 summarizes these findings using 2011 BRFSS data. District residents report being overweight or obese less frequently[2] than the U.S. residents overall. District residents also report greater engagement in exercise in the past 30 days. A greater percentage of older adults reported overweight and obesity and less "adequate" exercise compared to those 18–39 years old (Table 3.6). Despite better

Table 3.4
D.C. Adult Preventive Health Service Use by Ward Differences (percentage)

Variable	Ward 1	Ward 2	Ward 3	Ward 4	Ward 5	Ward 6	Ward 7	Ward 8
No routine checkup in the past year	27.0	21.9	29.3	21.1	17.6	23.9	16.3	15.8
No personal health care provider	17.2	12.8	13.1	11.3	21.4	10.7	17.1	15.2
Missed care in the last 12 months because of cost	4.5	6.7	4.8	8.0	10.4	8.0	12.5	16.1

SOURCE: 2010 BRFSS Annual Report; DOH, 2012.
NOTE: P-values are not provided because raw data were not accessible for analyses.

---

[2]   *Obesity* is defined as a body mass index (BMI) of 30.0 or greater. *Overweight* is defined as a BMI of 25.0–29.9.

Table 3.5
Adult Exercise and Obesity in D.C. Versus the United States

Variable	District of Columbia			United States			
	N	Percentage	SE	N	Percentage	SE	P-value
Exercise in the past 30 days	4,356	80.2	0.9	481,482	74.3	0.1	<.0.001
Inactive or insufficiently active over the past 30 days	4,152	42.6	1.2	461,191	48.9	0.2	<.0.001
Met aerobic recommendations	4,174	57.6	1.2	464,391	51.4	0.2	<.0.001
Met muscle strengthening recommendations	4,276	36.1	1.2	475,711	29.1	0.1	<.0.001
Obese	4,560	24.1	1.0	504,408	27.3	0.1	0.0010
Overweight or obese	4,560	53.2	1.2	504,408	63.2	0.1	<.0.001

SOURCE: BRFSS, 2011.

NOTE: N = total BRFSS sample. P-values in bold indicate that the difference between the United States and the District is statistically significant for p<0.05.

overall rates of obesity and exercise in the District, the racial/ethnic disparities are striking—a pattern that has persisted over the past decade (Table 3.7 and Figure 3.1). Black residents report being overweight or obese more frequently than white residents and report less vigorous exercise in the past month.

Differences in these health behaviors by ward were also notable, with a greater proportion of those in Wards 7 and 8 reporting no exercise in the past 30 days (30.6 percent and 31.5

Table 3.6
D.C. Adult Exercise and Obesity by Age

Variable	18–39 Years			40–64 Years			65 Years and Older			
	N	Percentage	SE	N	Percentage	SE	N	Percentage	SE	P-value
Exercise in the past 30 days	848	85.7	1.4	2,067	78.0	1.4	1,365	69.6	1.8	<.0001
Inactive or insufficiently active over the past 30 days	825	40.4	2.2	2,016	43.9	1.5	1,293	45.3	1.8	0.0324
Met aerobic recommendations	828	59.8	2.2	2,026	56.2	1.5	1,302	55.1	1.8	0.0389
Met muscle strengthening recommendations	829	42.6	2.3	2,035	32.3	1.3	1,337	26.5	1.4	<.0001
Obese	888	17.5	1.6	2,146	30.9	1.4	1,444	26.7	1.6	<.0001
Overweight or obese	888	42.9	2.1	2,146	62.3	1.4	1,444	61.3	1.6	<.0001

SOURCE: BRFSS, 2011.

NOTE: P-values in bold indicate that the difference between at least two age groups is statistically significant for p<0.05.

Table 3.7
D.C. Adult Exercise and Obesity by Race/Ethnicity

Variable	White, Non-Hispanic			Black, Non-Hispanic			
	N	Percentage	SE	N	Percentage	SE	P-value
Exercise in the past 30 days	1,945	91.4	0.8	1,910	71.8	1.6	<.0001
Inactive or insufficiently active over the past 30 days	1,892	29.8	1.5	1,795	51.6	1.9	<.0001
Met aerobic recommendations	1,898	70.2	1.5	1,807	48.8	1.9	<.0001
Met muscle strengthening recommendations	1,924	43.7	1.7	1,863	29.0	1.8	<.0001
Obese	1,998	11.0	1.1	2,034	36.8	1.7	<.0001
Overweight or obese	1,998	40.1	1.6	2,034	65.5	1.8	<.0001

SOURCE: BRFSS, 2011.

NOTE: N = total BRFSS sample. P-values in bold indicate that the difference between the black and white residents is statistically significant for p<0.05.

percent, respectively) compared to those in Ward 3, where 7.8 percent reported no exercise in the past 30 days. Obesity appears to be more common in Wards 7 and 8, while general overweight is more prevalent in Wards 4 and 5 (see Table 3.8). As noted earlier, testing of statistical significance could not be applied to ward comparisons.

We also examined patterns of nutrition, obesity, and overweight among youth, using 2011 YRBS data and comparing the District population to the U.S. population, as well as compar-

Figure 3.1
D.C. Adult Exercise and Obesity by Race/Ethnicity

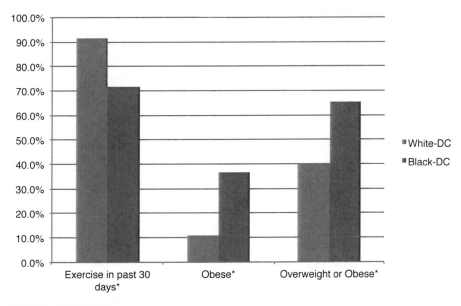

SOUREC: BRFSS, 2011.
NOTE: Asterisks indicate that the difference between the black and white residents is statistically significant for p<0.05.
RAND RR207-3.1

Table 3.8
D.C. Adult Overweight, Obesity, and Exercise by Ward (percentage)

Variable	Ward 1	Ward 2	Ward 3	Ward 4	Ward 5	Ward 6	Ward 7	Ward 8
Exercise in the past 30 days	83.7	86.0	92.2	79.9	72.4	85.1	69.4	68.5
Obese	21.3	14.4	7.5	25.8	29.9	17.4	35.3	44.4
Overweight	33.9	30.0	35.7	36.7	36.6	34.8	34.6	32.9

SOURCE: 2010 BRFSS Annual Report; DOH, 2012.

NOTE: P-values are not provided because raw data were not accessible for analyses.

ing patterns by gender. As shown in Table 3.9, District youth reported less frequent exercise in the past week, with nearly 72 percent reporting that they did not exercise at least 30 minutes per day for at least five days per week compared to 50 percent of youths nationally. Overall, self-reported obesity and overweight was more common among District youth, though gender differences were not significant. Nationally, the difference in self-reported obesity between boys and girls is statistically significant, with nearly twice as many boys reporting being obese than girls. Gender differences were notable in rates of physical activity, with girls reporting less exercise than boys (p<0.05) both in the District and nationally. Television viewing did not differ between the District and United States overall or between boys and girls in the District.

According to the National Survey of Children's Health, in 2007, 35.4 percent of children in the District aged 10–17 were overweight or obese as compared to 31.6 percent of children nationwide. Also, District children between the ages of 6 and 17 were less likely to have engaged in physical activity (defined as 20 minutes or more of activity causing them to sweat) during the prior week as compared to children in this age range nationally. Seventeen percent of District children between the ages of 4 and 17 reported no physical activity within the prior week as compared to 10.3 percent of children nationwide (Data Resource Center for Child and Adolescent Health, 2007).

Table 3.9
High School Student Exercise and Obesity in D.C. Versus the United States (percentage)

Variable	District of Columbia			United States		
	Total	Male	Female	Total	Male	Female
Physically active at least 30 minutes a day on less than 5 days per week	71.6	66.7*	75.8	50.5	40.1*	61.5
Watched television three or more hours a day	38.3	36.1	40.5	32.4	33.3	31.6
Overweight	18.0	16.4	19.5	15.2	15.1	15.4
Obese	14.5	13.4	15.5	13.0	16.1*	9.8

SOURCE: YRBS, 2011.

NOTE: P-values in bold indicate that the difference between the United States and the District is statistically significant for p<0.05; an asterisk indicates difference between males and females is significant at p<.05

Distribution of Fast Food Outlets and District Parks, Trails, and Bicycle Lanes

We also examined the location of fast-food outlets and places for exercise, including parks, trails, and bicycle lanes. Fast-food restaurants have been shown to be statistically significantly clustered in areas within short walking distance from schools, exposing children to poor-quality food environments in their school neighborhoods (Austin, 2005). Various studies have also found an association between the availability of places to exercise and rates of physical activity among youth. For example, neighborhoods with a greater proportion of park area are associated with greater physical activity in children aged 4–7 (Roemmich, 2006). Particular park features are also important to exercise patterns. Specifically, people are more likely to exercise at parks that have areas for moderate exercise, such as tracks, walking paths, and trails (Cohen, McKenzie, et al., 2007). Finally, the presence of bike lanes and sidewalks has also been shown to influence routine walking and cycling (Sallis and Owen, 1990; Giles-Corti and Donovan, 2003; De Bourdeaud Huij et al., 2003).

Figure 3.2 shows the distribution of major fast-food locations in the District, and Figure 3.3 shows a map of District parks, trails, and bicycle lanes. Many of the fast-food locations are concentrated in the center of the District, around Wards 1, 2, 5, and 6. The most developed trail systems in the area are generally found connecting wealthier suburbs with the city, such as the Capital Crescent Trail and the C&O Canal trail northwest of the city and the Mount Vernon Trail in Northern Virginia. Within the city, bicycle lanes are concentrated in downtown, and trails are concentrated in major parks like Rock Creek and the National Mall. In recent years, there has been a push to develop the trail systems in other areas of the city, such as the Anacostia Riverwalk Trail and the Marvin Gaye Park Trail in the east and the Metro-

Figure 3.2
Major Outlet Fast Food Locations

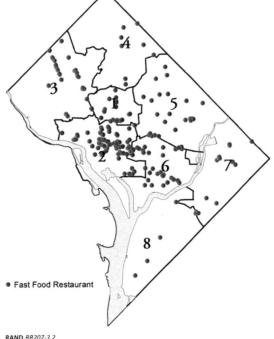

• Fast Food Restaurant

RAND *RR207-3.2*

Figure 3.3
District Parks, Trails, and Bicycle Lanes

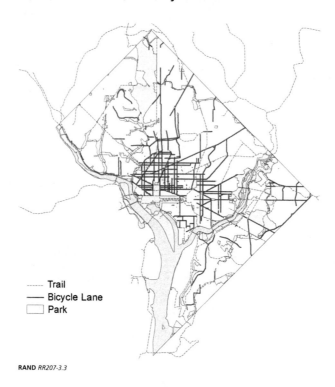

Trail
Bicycle Lane
Park

RAND *RR207-3.3*

politan Branch Trail in the north. This would open greater access to bike and walking trails for communities that may benefit from more exercise opportunities (e.g., Wards 7 and 8).

3.3 Chronic Disease and Disability

Examining rates of chronic disease and disability, there are some key differences between self-reported diagnoses in the District compared to the United States. First, fewer people in the District report ever being diagnosed with coronary heart disease, arthritis, and chronic obstructive pulmonary disorder (COPD). On the other hand, slightly more District residents report being diagnosed with asthma than do U.S. residents overall (16 percent versus 14 percent, $p<0.05$), and more District residents require special equipment due to health problems (11 percent versus 8 percent in the United States, $p<.001$).

The most common cancer among adult women is breast cancer, followed by lung and colorectal cancer. For men, prostate cancer is most prevalent, followed by lung and colorectal cancer. According to the most recent 2009 data, the age-adjusted incidence of prostate and pancreatic cancer was higher in the District than in the United States. Lung and skin cancer incidence is lower in the District than in the nation.

The incidence of pediatric cancer cases (all cancers among individuals younger than 20) is comparable in D.C. and nationwide. In the District, there were 14.8 cases of cancer (all cause) per 100,000 youths from 2005 to 2009 as compared to 16.9 cases per 100,000 youths nationwide. The difference is not statistically significant at $p<0.05$, possibly due to the small number of reported pediatric cancer cases in the District (National Cancer Institute, undated).

Table 3.10
Adult Chronic Disease and Disability in D.C. Versus the United States

Variable	District of Columbia			United States			
	N	Percentage	SE	N	Percentage	SE	P-value
Activity limited due to health problems	4,274	22.3	1.0	475,220	23.7	0.1	0.1648
Ever diagnosed with a heart attack	4,536	3.4	0.4	501,987	4.3	0.0	0.0123
Ever diagnosed with angina or coronary heart disease	4,522	3.0	0.3	499,809	4.3	0.0	0.0000
Ever diagnosed with arthritis	4,536	20.9	0.8	500,051	24.8	0.1	0.0000
Ever diagnosed with asthma	4,549	15.8	0.9	502,830	13.5	0.1	0.0065
Ever diagnosed with COPD	4,534	4.6	0.4	500,593	6.3	0.1	0.0001
Ever diagnosed with diabetes	4,551	9.1	0.6	502,486	9.8	0.1	0.2432
Ever diagnosed with kidney disease	4,545	2.7	0.3	501,585	2.5	0.0	0.6362
Ever diagnosed with stroke	4,547	3.7	0.3	503,031	2.9	0.0	0.0227
Ever diagnosed with vision or eye problems	4,487	16.4	0.8	497,557	19.9	0.1	0.0000
Special equipment due to health problems	4,289	10.8	0.6	476,922	7.9	0.1	0.0000
Still (currently) have asthma	4,528	10.1	0.7	501,119	8.8	0.1	0.0593

SOURCE: BRFSS, 2011.

NOTE: N = total BRFSS sample. P-values in bold indicate that the difference between the United States and the District is statistically significant for $p<0.05$.

Rates of adult chronic disease vary by age (Table 3.12). A greater percentage of older adults have angina or coronary heart disease, arthritics, and COPD. On the other hand, asthma prevalence is greater among those 18–39 and 40–64 years old.

While the overall District rates are favorable in terms of self-reported chronic illness, racial/ethnic disparities continue to be pronounced (Table 3.13). For example, more black residents than white residents report ever being diagnosed with angina or coronary heart disease, arthritis, asthma, and diabetes. Also, more black residents than white report activity limitations and the use of special equipment due to health problems. For cancer (not listed in Table 3.13), the age-adjusted incidence was 313.6 per 100,000 for white residents but 481.8 per 100,000 for black residents. The cancer rate for black residents is also higher in the District compared to the overall United States (473.1 per 100,000).

There are also differences in the rate of adult chronic disease and disability by ward (Table 3.14). More individuals in Ward 7 have been told they have cardiovascular disease and asthma compared to other wards. The prevalence of diabetes appeared highest in Ward 8, followed by Ward 5 and Ward 7. Limitations due to physical or emotional health were more frequently reported in Wards 7 and 8, followed by Wards 1 and 5.

According to the YRBS, approximately 30 percent of District high school students report that a doctor or nurse has told them they have asthma. This compares to about 23 percent of

Table 3.11
Age-Adjusted Incidence Rates per 100,000 for the Most Common Cancers in D.C. and the United States (2009)

Cancer Site	District of Columbia	United States
All cancer sites combined*	442.4	457.6
Prostate	166.9	137.1
Breast (female)*	130.9	122.8
Lung and bronchus	56.1	64.4
Colorectal	43.8	42.3
Uterine	23.5	24.0
Lymphomas	20.9	21.6
Pancreatic	15.9	11.7
Bladder	14.6	20.4
Skin (melanoma)	7.0	19.2
Oral cavity	10.3	10.9
Cervical	5.4	7.9

SOURCE: CDC WONDER, 2009.

NOTE: Values in bold indicate that the difference between the United States and the District is statistically significant for p<0.05.

* In situ breast cancers are not included in the breast or all sites categories. See also Price et al., 2012.

high school students nationally (Table 3.15). More boys in the District reported ever having been diagnosed with asthma than girls (p<0.05).

3.4 Reproductive and Sexual Health

Births and Infant Mortality

There were 9,156 births in the District in 2010, including 1,458 to mothers of Hispanic ethnicity (all races) and 4,940 to black mothers (DOH, 2012). Overall, the rate of preterm births (prior to 37 weeks gestation) in the District declined from 16.0 percent of all births in 2006 to 13.6 percent of all births in 2010 (Martin et al., 2012). Infant mortality in 2010 was at its lowest rate in a decade, having declined from 10.6 per 1,000 live births in 2001 to 8.0 per 1,000 live births in 2010. However, the District's 2010 rate was higher than the national rate of 6.1 per 1,000 live births during the same year. Also, significant disparities still exist by race and ward in D.C., with blacks having a rate of 10.7 per 1,000 live births as compared to a rate of 4.9 per 1,000 live births among whites and 3.7 per 1,000 live births among persons of Hispanic ethnicity in 2010. Rates were highest in Wards 4, 5, and 6 and lowest in Ward 2. Table 3.16 shows infant mortality rates by ward in the District. For that same year, rates of low birth weight (<2,500 grams) were highest in Wards 7 and 8 and lowest in Wards 3 and 4 (DOH, 2012).

Table 3.12
D.C. Adult Chronic Disease and Disability by Age

Variable	18–39 Years			40–64 Years			65 Years and Older			
	N	Percentage	SE	N	Percentage	SE	N	Percentage	SE	P-value
Activity limited due to health problems	829	13.1	1.7	2,023	28.0	1.4	1,346	35.5	1.7	<.0001
Ever diagnosed with a heart attack	885	0.7	0.5	2,136	3.5	0.5	1,434	10.6	1.3	<.0001
Ever diagnosed with angina or coronary heart disease	887	0.3	0.2	2,135	3.3	0.5	1,419	10.1	1.2	<.0001
Ever diagnosed with arthritis	884	5.5	1.0	2,135	26.3	1.3	1,436	53.0	1.7	<.0001
Ever diagnosed with asthma	887	16.1	1.6	2,139	16.8	1.1	1,441	12.6	1.2	0.0373
Ever diagnosed with COPD	883	2.0	0.6	2,137	6.3	0.7	1,432	8.1	1.0	<.0001
Ever diagnosed with diabetes	885	2.3	0.8	2,144	11.9	0.9	1,440	22.6	1.6	<.0001
Ever diagnosed with kidney disease	886	0.7	0.3	2,140	3.9	0.6	1,437	5.3	0.9	<.0001
Ever diagnosed with stroke	886	0.7	0.3	2,141	4.4	0.6	1,438	10.7	1.2	<.0001
Ever diagnosed with vision or eye problems	879	9.2	1.4	2,113	18.4	1.1	1,414	32.8	1.6	<.0001
Special equipment due to health problems	830	2.5	0.7	2,027	13.0	1.0	1,355	29.7	1.7	<.0001
Still (currently) have asthma	880	8.9	1.2	2,131	11.9	1.0	1,436	9.1	1.1	0.0059

SOURCE: BRFSS, 2011.

NOTE: N = total BRFSS sample. P-values in bold indicate that the difference between at least two age categories is statistically significant for p<0.05.

The number of births to mothers under the age of 20 declined by 8.5 percent from 1,057 in 2009 to 967 in 2010. The rate of births to mothers in this age range was highest in Wards 7 and 8 and lowest in Ward 4 (see table 3.16).

Sexually Transmitted Infections and HIV

D.C. continues to report high STI rates relative to the U.S. population. In 2010, the rate of reported chlamydia cases was 932 per 100,000 population (compared to the national rate of 426 per 100,000), the rate of reported gonorrhea cases was 350.9 per 100,000 population (compared to the national rate of 100.8 per 100,000), and the rate of reported syphilis cases was 22.3 per 100,000 population (compared to the national rate of 4.5 per 100,000) (CDC, 2010, Sexually Transmitted Disease Surveillance). By ward over a five-year period, rates of aggregate chlamydia and gonorrhea cases were highest in Wards 7 and 8 and lowest in Ward 3

Table 3.13
D.C. Adult Chronic Disease and Disability by Race/Ethnicity

Variable	White, Non-Hispanic			Black, Non-Hispanic			
	N	Percentage	SE	N	Percentage	SE	P-value
Activity limited due to health problems	1,922	16.6	1.1	1,867	27.7	1.6	<.0001
Ever diagnosed with a heart attack	1,994	1.2	0.3	2,019	4.9	0.7	<.0001
Ever diagnosed with angina or coronary heart disease	1,985	1.9	0.3	2,013	3.6	0.5	0.0011
Ever diagnosed with arthritis	1,988	13.9	0.8	2,025	27.9	1.4	<.0001
Ever diagnosed with asthma	1,994	12.7	1.1	2,028	18.4	1.4	<.0001
Ever diagnosed with COPD	1,989	2.1	0.4	2,023	6.8	0.8	<.0001
Ever diagnosed with diabetes	1,997	2.8	0.4	2,030	15.0	1.1	<.0001
Ever diagnosed with kidney disease	1,993	1.3	0.3	2,031	3.8	0.5	<.0001
Ever diagnosed with stroke	1,994	1.2	0.2	2,027	5.5	0.6	<.0001
Ever diagnosed with vision or eye problems	1,967	13.1	1.0	2,004	18.4	1.2	<.0001
Special equipment due to health problems	1,925	4.7	0.5	1,874	16.4	1.1	<.0001
Still (currently) have asthma	1,990	6.1	0.8	2,016	13.3	1.2	<.0001

SOURCE: BRFSS, 2011.

NOTE: N = total BRFSS sample. P-values in bold indicate that the difference between the black and white residents is statistically significant for p<0.05.

(see Table 3.17). The rate of primary and secondary syphilis cases were highest in Wards 1 and 2 and lowest in Ward 3 over that same period (DOH, 2011).

Hepatitis B and C are also of concern in the District and are commonly present as coinfections with each other or as coinfections with HIV. About 19 percent of individuals in the District with chronic hepatitis B also have HIV, and 14.9 percent of individuals with chronic hepatitis B are coinfected with chronic hepatitis C. Rates of chronic hepatitis B are highest in Ward 1 (five-year aggregate rate of 336 per 100,000 individuals) and rates of chronic hepatitis

Table 3.14
D.C. Adult Chronic Disease and Disability by Ward (percentage)

Variable	Ward 1	Ward 2	Ward 3	Ward 4	Ward 5	Ward 6	Ward 7	Ward 8
Currently have asthma	6.8	9.0	8.5	10.5	15.7	11.4	17.5	10.7
Ever told they had cardiovascular disease	1.5	1.2	2.0	2.2	2.4	2.9	4.8	3.6
Ever told they have diabetes	7.1	6.1	2.2	10.2	12.5	6.7	11.6	15.2
Limitations due to physical or emotional health	19.5	12.8	17.4	15.8	18.6	15.8	21.7	21.2

SOURCE: 2010 BRFSS Annual Report; DOH, 2012.

NOTE: P-values are not provided because raw data were not accessible for analyses.

Table 3.15
High School Student Asthma Rates in D.C. Versus the United States (percentage)

Variable	District of Columbia			United States		
	Total	Male	Female	Total	Male	Female
Ever told by a doctor or nurse they had asthma	29.5	33.1[b]	26.1	23.0	23.2	22.8
Ever told by a doctor or nurse they had asthma and current asthma[a]	—	—	—	11.9	10.4	13.5

SOURCE: YRBS, 2011.

NOTE: P-values in bold indicate that the difference between the United States and the District is statistically significant for p<0.05.

[a] Data are not available for 2011 (or even 2009) for this question in D.C.

[b] Indicates that the difference between males and females is significant at p<0.05.

C are highest in Ward 8 (five-year aggregate rate of 2,150 per 100,000 individuals), as shown in Table 3.17 (DOH, 2011).

In 2010, the number of newly diagnosed cases of HIV (including AIDS) was 835, down from 1,103 in 2006. The majority of new cases were from sexual contact. Of the new cases in 2010, 305 (36.5 percent) were from men having sex with men, 278 (33.3 percent) were from heterosexual intercourse, 42 (5 percent) were from injection drug use (IDU), 15 (1.8 percent) were from a mixture of men having sex with men and IDU, and 195 (23.4 percent) were from unidentified causes. Of the 835 new cases in 2010, 648 (78 percent) occurred among blacks (DOH, 2011). Deaths related to HIV (including AIDS) declined in 2010 to 207 from 399 in 2006. However, the death rate among black men remained steady over the previous five years (DOH, 2011).

Sexual Health Infection Testing and Prevention

Nearly two times as many adults in the District received an HIV test in their lifetime than in the United States overall (Table 3.18). This translates to almost 68 percent of people in the District over the age of 18 reporting ever having an HIV test as compared to just over 37 percent of the general U.S. population. Testing is most prevalent among those aged 18–39 years (Table 3.19). In addition, more black adult residents of the District report having an HIV test compared to white adult residents (Table 3.20). Ward differences in HIV testing rates indicate the most reported testing in Wards 7 and 8 and the least reports of testing in Ward 3 (Table 3.21). Additionally, Ward 8 reported a greater use of condoms at last intercourse as compared

Table 3.16
D.C. Rates of Infant Mortality, Low Birth Weight, and Births to Mothers Under Age 20 by Ward (per 1,000 live births)

Variable	All	Ward 1	Ward 2	Ward 3	Ward 4	Ward 5	Ward 6	Ward 7	Ward 8
Infant mortality	8.0	4.1	2.9	5.0	11.3	10.3	9.8	6.6	10.4
Low birth weight	10.2	9.3	5.8	5.7	8.8	11.3	10.2	12.9	13.4
Births mothers under age 20	10.6	7.3	2.9	0.2	8.6	11.9	6.1	18.3	18.3

SOURCE: Department of Health, Data Management and Analysis Division, Center for Policy, Planning and Evaluation, *2010 Infant Mortality Rate for the District of Columbia*, April 26, 2012.

Table 3.17
D.C. Five-Year Aggregate Rates of Chlamydia, Gonorrhea, Syphilis, and Chronic Hepatitis B and C by Ward (per 100,000 population)

STI	Ward 1	Ward 2	Ward 3	Ward 4	Ward 5	Ward 6	Ward 7	Ward 8
Chlamydia	549.9	224.0	80.4	504.1	979.7	531.3	1,348.0	1,770.6
Gonorrhea	207.4	148.9	18.2	146.5	378.2	241.5	505.2	739.6
Syphilis (primary and secondary)	38.1	35.0	1.3	11.9	21.5	17.0	29.5	19.8
Chronic hepatitis B	336	258	93	327	322	287	277	329
Chronic hepatitis C	965	529	156	880	1,488	1,270	1,699	2,150

SOURCE: District of Columbia Department of Health, *HIV/AIDS, Hepatitis, STD, and TB Epidemiology in the District of Columbia*, 2011.

NOTE: Cases for which ward information was available, including cases diagnosed in jail and for homeless individuals.

Table 3.18
Adult HIV Testing in D.C. Versus the United States

	District of Columbia			United States			
Variable	N	Percentage	SE	N	Percentage	SE	P-value
Ever had an HIV test (18 years and older)	4,106	67.9	1.1	453,385	37.4	0.2	**0.0000**

SOURCE: BRFSS, 2011.

NOTE: N = total BRFSS sample. P-values in bold indicate that the difference between the United States and the District is statistically significant for p<0.05.

Table 3.19
D.C. Adult HIV Testing by Age

	18–39 Years			40–64 Years			65 Years and Older			
Variable	N	Percentage	SE	N	Percentage	SE	N	Percentage	SE	P-value
Ever had an HIV test	809	73.2	2.2	1,954	73.9	1.3	1,273	36.0	1.8	**<.0001**

SOURCE: BRFSS, 2011.

NOTE: N = total BRFSS sample. P-values in bold indicate that the difference between at least two age groups is statistically significant for p<0.05.

Table 3.20
D.C. Adult HIV Testing by Race/Ethnicity Differences

	White, Non-Hispanic			Black, Non-Hispanic			P-value
Variable	N	Percentage	SE	N	Percentage	SE	
Ever had an HIV test (18 years and older)	1,838	59.4	1.7	1,796	75.5	1.6	**<.0001**

SOURCE: BRFSS, 2011.

NOTE: N = total BRFSS sample. P-values in bold indicate that the difference between the black and white residents is statistically significant for p<0.05.

Table 3.21
D.C. Adult Reproductive and Sexual Health by Ward (percentage)

Variable	Ward 1	Ward 2	Ward 3	Ward 4	Ward 5	Ward 6	Ward 7	Ward 8
Ever had an HIV test (18 years and older)	66.8	69.7	61.8	70.1	74.9	71.5	76.6	81.8
Use of condom during last intercourse	40.3	40.2	30.3	33.1	45.1	29.0	47.1	48.1
Treated for an STI in the past 12 months	2.3	3.6	1.0	1.8	5.0	1.5	14.5	8.6

SOURCE: 2010 BRFSS Annual Report; DOH, 2012.

NOTE: P-values are not provided because raw data were not accessible for analyses.

to other wards. Ward 7 noted the highest reported prevalence of STI treatment during the last 12 months as compared to other wards.

Youth Sexual Behavior

In 2011, 55 percent of District high school students reported ever having sexual intercourse (compared to 47 percent of youth nationally) (Table 3.22). Early sexual intercourse (before 13 years of age) is more common in the District than in the nation as a whole (13 percent versus 6 percent). About 13 percent of District youth report not using any form of pregnancy prevention at last intercourse (compared to a similar percentage nationally). There was no difference in the percentage of youth who reported using alcohol at last intercourse (22.9 percent in the District versus 22.1 percent in the United States).

Table 3.22
High School Student Sexual and Reproductive Health in D.C. Versus the United States (percentage)

Variable	District of Columbia			United States		
	Total	Male	Female	Total	Male	Female
Ever had sexual intercourse	54.9	61.7*	49.3	47.4	49.2	45.6
Sexual intercourse before age 13	13.3	24.0*	4.6	6.2	9.0*	3.4
Did not use contraception at last intercourse	13.4	11.3	15.3	12.9	10.6*	15.1
Alcohol use at last intercourse	22.9	25.8	19.7	22.1	26.0*	18.1

SOURCE: YRBS, 2011.

* Indicates that the difference between males and females is significant at p<0.05.

Table 3.23
Number and Percentage of Chlamydia and Gonorrhea Cases Among D.C. Youth Aged 15–19 (2006–2010)

STI	2006	2007	2008	2009	2010
Chlamydia					
Ages 15–19 n (percent)	1,239 (36.9)	2,215 (36.7)	2,694 (39.0)	2,610 (39.7)	2,351 (42.0)
Total cases n	3,360	6,042	6,899	6,568	5,592
Gonorrhea					
Ages 15–19 n (percent)	495 (26.4)	638 (26.9)	880 (33.3)	871 (33.9)	743 (35.3)
Total cases n	1,877	2,375	2,646	2,567	2,104

SOURCE: District of Columbia Department of Health, *HIV/AIDS, Hepatitis, STD, and TB Epidemiology.*

3.5 Mental Health and Substance Use

Mental Health

According to data from the 2010 and 2011 National Surveys of Drug Use and Health, 22.6 percent of District adults over the age of 18 reported any mental illness as compared to 19.83 percent of adults nationwide, although the difference is not statistically significant (SAMHSA, 2010–2011).

The rate of diagnosis of depressive disorder among adults also appears to be comparable to U.S. reports (2010 BRFSS), although fewer people in the District report having necessary social or emotional support (asked as "do you feel you have enough social or emotional sup-

Table 3.24
Adult Mental Health and Substance Use in D.C. Versus the United States

Variable	District of Columbia			United States			P-value
	N	Percentage	SE	N	Percentage	SE	
Current smoker	4,518	20.8	1.0	501,876	20.1	0.1	0.5002
Ever a smoker	4,518	42.8	1.1	501,876	44.8	0.1	0.0848
Smokers stopped in the last 12 months	688	62.9	2.9	83,934	59.5	0.3	0.2437
Binge drinking	4,210	25.0	1.2	467,758	18.3	0.1	**0.0000**
Heavy drinking	4,216	9.6	0.8	467,520	6.6	0.1	**0.0002**
Ever diagnosed with depressive disorder	4,534	16.0	0.8	500,980	16.8	0.1	0.3484
Always receive necessary social support*	3,699	45.2	1.0	425,545	51.3	0.2	**0.0000**

SOURCE: BRFSS, 2011.

NOTE: N=total BRFSS sample. P-values in bold indicate that the difference between the United States and the District is statistically significant for p<0.05.

* Only asked in the 2010 BRFSS.

port?") compared to the overall United States (51 percent). Diagnosis of depressive disorder was more common among those 40–64 years old than among other age groups.

According to a 2010 report about behavioral health care in the District, there is significant unmet need for persons with mental illness, particularly those covered by Medicaid managed care or DC Alliance and those who lack insurance. Approximately 60 percent of adults and 72 percent of adolescents enrolled in a Medicaid managed care plan were estimated to have an unmet need for depression care (Gresenz, 2010).

District youth have lower rates of feelings of sadness compared to the rest of the country, with 23 percent of District high school students reporting feeling sad of hopeless for at least two weeks in the past 30 days compared to 28 percent of youth nationally. Also, a greater proportion of youth nationally seriously considered suicide (16 percent) compared to District youth (12 percent) (p<0.05).

Smoking and Substance Abuse

Binge drinking and heavy drinking is more common in the District than in the overall United States. By age group, more 18–39-year-olds report binge and heavy drinking (39 percent binge; 13 percent heavy) and more 40–64-year-olds report being current smokers (Table 3.25) than other age groups (23 percent versus 11 percent of those 65 years and older and 21 percent of 18–39-year-olds). There are also racial differences in substance use (Figure 3.4). More white residents than black residents report frequent engagement in binge drinking (32 percent white versus 18 percent black) and heavy drinking (12 percent white versus 7 percent black).

Despite low overall rates of smoking in the District, it is more commonly reported in Wards 5 and 8 (Table 3.26). Heavy drinking is more prevalent in Wards 3 and 6, though statistical testing could not be applied.

The District has higher rates of illicit drug use among all ages (12 and above) as compared to the United States overall, with 13.5 percent of District residents reporting any illicit drug use

Table 3.25
D.C. Adult Mental Health and Substance Use by Age

Variable	18–39 years			40–64 years			65 years and older			
	N	Percentage	SE	N	Percentage	SE	N	Percentage	SE	P-value
Current smoker	882	22.2	1.9	2,127	23.1	1.3	1,428	11.0	1.2	**<.0001**
Ever a smoker	882	34.0	2.1	2,127	48.3	1.5	1,428	54.8	1.7	**<.0001**
Smokers stopped in the last 12 months	149	59.5	5.0	395	66.4	3.3	133	63.7	5.4	0.2081
Binge drinking	813	39.0	2.2	2,000	16.9	1.2	1,327	5.4	0.7	**<.0001**
Heavy drinking	815	13.1	1.6	2,002	7.0	0.7	1,328	5.6	0.7	**<.0001**
Ever diagnosed with depressive disorder	884	13.4	1.5	2,134	20.3	1.2	1,434	12.9	1.1	**<.0001**
Always receive necessary social support*	732	44.1	2.2	1,764	42.1	1.4	1,157	51.2	1.7	**<.0001**

SOURCE: BRFSS, 2011.

NOTE: N=total BRFSS sample. P-values in bold indicate that the difference between any two age groups is statistically significant for p<0.05.

Figure 3.4
D.C. Adult Substance Use by Race/Ethnicity

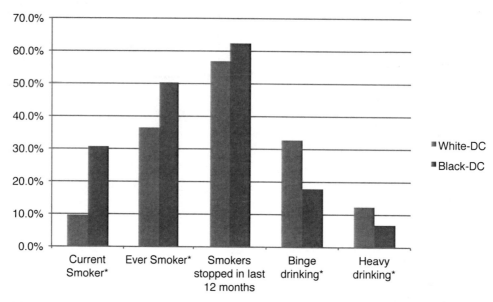

SOUREC: BRFSS, 2011.
NOTE: Asterisks indicate that the difference between black and white residents is statistically significant for p<0.05.
RAND RR207-3.4

in the past 30 days compared to 8.8 percent of residents nationwide (p<0.05). About 18.5 percent of District residents used marijuana in the past 30 days as compared to 11.6 percent of residents nationwide (p<0.05), and about 3 percent of District residents used cocaine in the past year as compared to 1.6 percent of residents nationwide (p<0.05). District residents reported nonmedical use of prescription drugs in the past year at rates similar to residents nationwide (4.7 percent versus 4.6 percent in the United States) (SAMHSA, 2011).

In 2011, 13 percent of District high school students reporting having five or more drinks in one day (binge drinking) compared to 22 percent of youth nationally (p<0.05). However, though the rates are not significantly different, more District high school students reported using marijuana one or more times in the last 30 days than youth nationally (26 percent versus

Table 3.26
D.C. Adult Emotional Health and Substance Use by Ward (percentage)

Variable	Ward 1	Ward 2	Ward 3	Ward 4	Ward 5	Ward 6	Ward 7	Ward 8
Always obtain necessary emotional and social support	44.8	42.0	42.9	43.2	43.4	43.0	51.6	46.6
Current smoker	10.7	8.3	8.5	8.9	23.0	15.4	22.3	29.7
Ever a smoker	39.2	34.2	38.7	35.6	42.1	40.6	41.0	44.4
Binge drinking	17.9	18.8	16.7	14.6	10.4	20.0	6.2	11.9
Heavy drinking	5.2	6.4	8.6	4.1	3.4	7.8	2.4	5.5

SOURCE: 2010 BRFSS Annual Report; DOH, 2012.

NOTE: P-values are not provided because raw data were not accessible for analyses.

23 percent). Cigarette use is more common among youth nationally, with 18 percent reporting smoking on at least one day in the past 30 days compared to 12 percent of District youth (p<0.05) (see Table 3.27).

Distribution of Alcohol Outlets

To further contextualize the binge drinking rates, we examined the location of alcohol outlets. The density of establishments selling alcohol for consumption off premises has been linked to the risk of injuries among children from accidents, assaults, and child abuse (Freisthler et al., 2008). In addition, the density of off-premise alcohol retail establishments has been shown to be associated with rates of violence and assault in particular (Gruenewald et al., 2006).

Figure 3.5 shows the distribution of alcohol outlets in the District using alcohol licensing data. Wards 7 and 8 have more liquor and grocery store alcohol outlets relative to restaurant alcohol outlets as compared to wards west of the Anacostia River, though binge drinking and heavy drinking is much higher in other wards. It is unclear if those outlets are used by residents in other wards or if these outlets simply do not contribute to heavy drinking in Wards 7 and 8. However, we did not assess the prevalence of accidents and other injuries, which could be correlated with the higher concentration of alcohol outlets.

3.6 Oral Health

Oral Health Among Adults

Oral health is an increasing problem nationally, and the District is no exception. More residents in the District have had a tooth removed due to decay compared to the general U.S. population (48 percent versus 45 percent, p<.001). However, a higher rate of District residents also report having their teeth professionally cleaned in the past year compared to the entire nation (73 percent versus 69 percent, p<.001) (Table 3.28).

Older adults report more tooth removal due to decay compared to those 18–39 years old, and dental visits are more common among the 18–39 age group (Table 3.29). Racial/

Table 3.27
High School Student Mental Health and Substance Use in D.C. Versus the United States (percentage)

Variable	District of Columbia			United States		
	Total	Male	Female	Total	Male	Female
Binge drinking in the last 30 days	**12.6**	12.2	12.9	**21.9**	23.8*	19.8
Marijuana use in the last 30 days	26.1	28.5	24.0	23.1	25.9*	20.1
Smoked at least one day in last 30 days	**12.5**	15.3*	9.3	**18.1**	19.9*	16.1
Feeling sad or hopeless in the last two weeks	24.9	21.0*	28.1	28.5	21.5*	35.9
Considered suicide	**11.1**	9.3	12.4	**15.8**	12.5*	19.3

SOURCE: YRBS, 2011.

NOTE: P-values in bold indicate that the difference between the US and the District is statistically significant for p<0.05.

* Indicates that the difference between males and females is significant at p<0.05.

Figure 3.5
Alcohol Outlets in the District

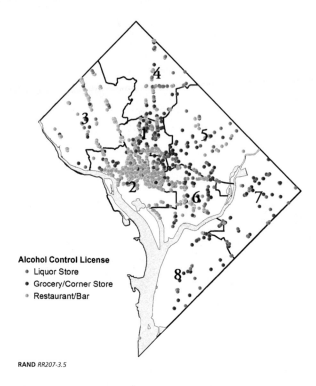

Alcohol Control License
- Liquor Store
- Grocery/Corner Store
- Restaurant/Bar

RAND *RR207-3.5*

ethnic disparities also exist, with more black residents noting the removal of any teeth due to decay than white residents (64 percent versus 29 percent, p<.0001), which is perhaps partially explained by the stark difference in reports of dental cleaning. Only 61 percent of black residents report having their teeth professionally cleaned in the past year compared to 87 percent of white residents (p<.0001) (Table 3.30).

Table 3.28
Adult Oral Health in D.C. Versus the United States

Variable	District of Columbia			United States			
	N	Percentage	SE	N	Percentage	SE	P-value
All teeth removed due to decay	3,888	3.9	0.4	442,397	4.9	0.0	**0.0073**
Any teeth removed due to decay	3,888	48.2	1.0	442,397	45.5	0.2	**0.0051**
Have not visited a dentist in five or more years	3,956	7.8	0.5	447,666	10.9	0.1	**0.0000**
Teeth not professionally cleaned in five or more years	3,788	7.7	0.6	405,393	10.7	0.1	**0.0000**
Teeth professionally cleaned in the past two years	3,788	83.6	0.8	405,393	80.0	0.1	**0.0000**
Teeth professionally cleaned in the past year	3,788	73.0	0.9	405,393	68.5	0.2	**0.0000**

SOURCE: BRFSS, 2011.

NOTE: N = total BRFSS sample. P-values in bold indicate that the difference between the United States and the District is statistically significant for p<0.05.

Table 3.29
D.C. Adult Oral Health by Age

Variable	18–39 years			40–64 years			65 years and older			P-value
	N	Percentage	SE	N	Percentage	SE	N	Percentage	SE	
All teeth removed due to decay	882	0.1	0.1	2,127	1.8	0.3	1,428	11.0	1.2	**<.0001**
Any teeth removed due to decay	882	34.0	2.1	2,127	48.3	1.5	1,428	54.8	1.7	**<.0001**
Have not visited a dentist in five or more years	149	6.0	1.0	395	6.6	0.7	133	11.6	1.2	0.2081
Teeth not professionally cleaned in five or more years	813	7.4	1.2	2,000	7.1	0.8	1,327	8.9	1.1	**<.0001**
Teeth professionally cleaned in the past two years	815	13.1	1.6	2,002	7.0	0.7	1,328	5.6	0.7	**<.0001**
Teeth professionally cleaned in the past year	884	13.4	1.5	2,134	20.3	1.2	1,434	12.9	1.1	**<.0001**
All teeth removed due to decay	732	44.1	2.2	1,764	42.1	1.4	1,157	51.2	1.7	**<.0001**

SOURCE: BRFSS, 2011.

NOTE: N=total BRFSS sample. P-values in bold indicate that the difference between at least two age groups is statistically significant for p<0.05.

Table 3.30
D.C. Adult Oral Health by Race/Ethnicity

Variable	White, Non-Hispanic			Black, Non-Hispanic			P-value
	N	Percentage	SE	N	Percentage	SE	
All teeth removed due to decay	1,885	0.9	0.2	1,572	7.0	0.7	**<.0001**
Any teeth removed due to decay	1,885	29.1	1.1	1,572	63.8	1.5	**<.0001**
Have not visited a dentist in five or more years	1,909	2.6	0.4	1,608	12.3	1.0	**<.0001**
Teeth not professionally cleaned in five or more years	1,891	3.3	0.6	1,469	11.9	1.0	**<.0001**
Teeth professionally cleaned in the past two years	1,891	92.9	0.7	1,469	75.1	1.4	**<.0001**
Teeth professionally cleaned in the past year	1,891	86.9	0.9	1,469	61.4	1.5	**<.0001**

SOURCE: BRFSS, 2011.

NOTE: N=total BRFSS sample. P-values in bold indicate that the difference between black and white residents is significant for p<0.05.

Table 3.31
D.C. Adult Oral Health by Ward (percentage)

Variable	Ward 1	Ward 2	Ward 3	Ward 4	Ward 5	Ward 6	Ward 7	Ward 8
Been to a dentist for any reason in the past year	67.5	87.0	88.3	71.3	66.3	79.2	63.1	60.4
Had at least one tooth removed due to decay	33.8	32.9	26.5	42.7	53.3	34.1	56.8	60.3
Had teeth cleaned in the past year	67.5	85.7	85.0	74.2	63.6	79.5	63.8	53.3

SOURCE: BRFSS, 2011.

NOTE: N = total BRFSS sample.

Ward differences are also pronounced, though these data are not analyzed by the RAND study and thus not adjusted for race/ethnicity and other factors. More residents in Wards 2 and 3 (87 percent and 88 percent, respectively) report visiting a dentist for any reason in the past year, as well as more frequent cleaning (86 percent and 85 percent, respectively) than residents in other wards. On the other hand, more residents in Wards 8, 7, and 5 note having a tooth removed due to decay than residents in other wards.

Child Oral Health

Less data are available about oral health care for children in the District. District children have rates of tooth decay and cavities similar to children nationwide. In 2007, about 19.8 percent of District parents of children aged 1–17 reported that their child had at least one cavity or decayed tooth in the prior six months as compared to 19.4 percent of parents nationwide (Data Resource Center for Child and Adolescent Health, 2007).

The overall level of oral health care among low-income children in D.C. is low but consistent with that nationwide. According to the Centers for Medicare and Medicaid Services (CMS), from 2000 to 2009, the national percentage of children under the age of 20 enrolled in Medicaid or the Children's Health Insurance Program (CHIP) who were receiving any dental service increased from 27 percent to 40 percent. In the District, there was a comparable increase from 23 percent to 40 percent among children covered by Medicaid (in D.C., CHIP is integrated into Medicaid) during this same time period. The District rate for preventive care visits for children enrolled in Medicaid/CHIP is higher than that nationwide (CMS, 2011).

3.7 Injuries

The BRFSS examines the extent to which adults are engaged in injury prevention behaviors (e.g., wearing a seat belt) and summarizes injury data related to falls for older adults. Other injury data were not available from this source.

There were no significant differences in these outcomes between District residents and U.S. residents (Table 3.32). More white residents reported using a seat belt than black residents. There are no major differences in falls for those between the ages of 40 and 64 and those who

Table 3.32
Adult Injuries in D.C. Versus the United States

| Variable | District of Columbia | | | United States | | | |
	N	Percentage	SE	N	Percentage	SE	P-value
Any falls in the past three months (age 45 and older)*	2,834	16.0	0.8	336,702	15.7	0.1	0.7144
Any falls in the past three months with injury (age 45 and older)*	2,834	5.5	0.5	336,577	5.3	0.1	0.7037
Always wear seatbelt	4,283	86.1	1.0	475,435	86.9	0.1	0.4415

SOURCE: BRFSS, 2011.

NOTE: N = total BRFSS sample. P-values in bold indicate that the difference between the United States and the District is statistically significant for p<0.05.

* Only asked in the 2010 BRFSS.

are 65 and older (Table 3.33). However, more white residents over the age of 45 reported falls in the past three months compared to black residents (Table 3.34).

Adults in Ward 5 were more likely to report falls compared to adults in other wards according to data from 2010 (8.5 percent reported falling 2 to 3 times in the past three months). Adults in Ward 8 were the least likely to use seat belts (13 percent) followed by those in Ward 1 (12 percent).

The YRBS queries youth about unintentional injuries and aggressive or violent behaviors ("intentional" injury). As shown in Table 3.35, more District high school students reported never using a seat belt (11 percent) compared to youth nationally (8 percent). There was no difference between the U.S. rates and the District rates in terms of carrying a weapon on school property, and fewer District youth reported being bullied at school (10 percent) compared to the U.S. average of 20 percent. On the other hand, more high school youth in the District reported physical abuse in intimate relationships (e.g., boyfriend/girlfriend) (15 percent versus 9 percent in the United States overall).

The District has a higher violent crime rate as compared to the rest of the country, with 1,202.1 violent crimes per 100,000 population versus the national rate of 386.3 per 100,000 in 2011. The murder rate was also higher, with 17.5 murders per 100,000 residents in 2011 compared to 4.7 murders per 100,000 nationwide. The aggravated assault rate is 494.3 per 100,000 population in the District as compared to 241.1 per 100,000 nationwide (Federal Bureau of Investigation, undated). The District has observed a downward trend in its homicide rate, which reached a 20-year low in 2012, when the number of homicides was 88 compared to 243 in 2003 and 454 in 1993 (District of Columbia Metropolitan Police Department, 2013).

3.8 Summary

Our analysis of health need suggests some important findings across the seven domain areas, which we briefly summarize in this section.

Table 3.33
D.C. Adult Injuries by Age

Variable	18–39 Years			40–64 Years			65 Years and Older			
	N	Percentage	SE	N	Percentage	SE	N	Percentage	SE	P-value
Any falls in the past three months (age 45 and older)*	0	—	—	1,212	16.0	1.1	2,774	16.4	1.3	0.7731
Any falls in the past three months with injury (age 45 and older)*	0	—	—	1,212	6.0	0.8	2,774	5.0	0.7	0.2575
Always wear seatbelt	829	82.7	1.9	2,027	88.5	1.1	1,350	89.9	1.0	**<.0001**

SOURCE: BRFSS, 2011.

NOTE: N=total BRFSS sample. P-values in bold indicate that the difference between at least two age groups is statistically significant for p<0.05.

* Only asked in the 2010 BRFSS.

General Health and the Use of Preventive Services

Overall, the use of preventive health services is better in the District than in the overall United States, with the percentage of adults who did not have a routine health care visit in the prior year and who did not report a regular provider lower than those nationwide. There is significant variability by ward, with Ward 1 having the highest percentage of individuals who reported no routine medical visit in the prior year and Ward 5 having the highest percentage of individuals without a regular provider. Ward 8 has the highest percentage of persons reporting difficulty seeing a provider in the prior year due to cost. More 18–39- and 40–64-year-olds missed care due to cost compared to those 65 years and older.

Nutrition and Obesity

District residents are also more likely to report exercise in the prior month than U.S. residents overall. However, black residents have a significantly higher rate of overweight and obesity than white residents. Overweight and obesity is highest among those forty years old and older, and self-reported rates of getting enough exercise are lowest among older adults.

Table 3.34
D.C. Adult Injuries by Race/Ethnicity

Variable	White, Non-Hispanic			Black, Non-Hispanic			
	N	Percentage	SE	N	Percentage	SE	P-value
Any falls in the past three months (age 45 and older)*	1,358	17.4	1.2	1,209	14.1	1.2	**0.0221**
Any falls in the past three months with injury (age 45 and older)*	1,358	4.7	0.6	1,209	6.3	0.9	0.1017
Always wear seatbelt	1,930	88.9	1.2	1,863	84.9	1.5	**0.0003**

SOURCE: BRFSS, 2011.

NOTE: N=total BRFSS sample. P-values in bold indicate that the difference between the black and white residents is statistically significant for p<0.05.

* Only asked in the 2010 BRFSS.

Table 3.35
High School Student Injuries in D.C. Versus the United States (percentage)

Variable	District of Columbia			United States		
	Total	Male	Female	Total	Male	Female
Rarely or never wear a seat belt	10.9	13.1*	8.3	7.7	8.9*	6.3
Carried a weapon on school property at least once in the past 30 days	5.5	8.2*	3.1	5.4	8.2*	2.3
Bullied on school property	**9.7**	12.2*	7.1	**20.1**	18.2*	22.0
In a physical fight one or more times in the last 30 days	37.9	42.2*	33.5	32.8	40.7*	24.4
Hit, slapped, or physically hurt by boyfriend/girlfriend	**14.7**	15.5	13.6	**9.4**	9.5	9.3

SOURCE: BRFSS, 2011.

NOTE: N = total BRFSS sample. P-values in bold indicate that the difference between the United States and the District is statistically significant for p<0.05.

* Indicates that the difference between males and females is significant at p<0.05.

Chronic Disease and Disability

The reported percentages of District residents with coronary heart disease, arthritis, and COPD are lower than those nationwide, but rates of asthma are higher. Again, disparities exist by race, with blacks having higher rates of heart disease, arthritis, COPD, and asthma. Blacks also have considerably higher rates of cancer than whites in the District, as well as nationwide. Perhaps not surprisingly, arthritis is greatest among those 65 and older, as is COPD. However, being ever diagnosed with depressive disorder is greatest among those 40–64 years old.

Reproductive and Sexual Health

The infant mortality rate in the District has declined significantly in the past ten years. The number of newly diagnosed HIV (including AIDS) cases has also declined in the past five years, as have deaths from HIV (including AIDS). While the majority of new cases were among blacks, the death rate among blacks has remained constant over this time. District residents report higher rates of HIV testing compared to the rest of the country, and those rates are highest among those 18–39 years old. D.C. continues to report high rates of gonorrhea and chlamydia as compared to the rest of the country, with rates particularly high in Wards 7 and 8. Youth in the District have a higher rate of sexual activity compared to youth nationally. Also, youth ages 15–19 have accounted for an increase in the proportion of chlamydia and gonorrhea cases in the city over the past five years.

Mental Health and Substance Use

Rates of depressive disorders are lower in the District than nationwide, with blacks reporting lower rates than whites. Fewer individuals aged 40 and above (compared to 18–39-year-olds) report that they always or usually receive necessary emotional or social support. Binge drinking and heavy drinking are more common in the District than across the overall United States. Binge and heavy drinking is more common among 18–39-year-olds than among other age groups. Current smoking is less prevalent among those 65 and older, though rates of having ever been a smoker follow the age pattern, with increasing experience with smoking consistent with increasing age.

Oral Health

A higher percentage of residents in the District have had a tooth removed due to decay than across the United States; however, more District residents also report having their teeth cleaned as compared to residents nationwide. Rates of any dental visit, as well as preventive care dental visits, specifically among children covered by Medicaid, are low in the District, but comparable to the national average. The rate of having any teeth removed increases with age, with nearly 70 percent of those 65 years and older reporting that experience.

Injuries

District residents engage in injury prevention behaviors at a similar rate to the rest of the country; however, black residents report a lower rate of seat belt use compared to white residents. White residents are also more likely to report falls than black residents. There is no variance by age group of adults who report seat belt use, and there is no difference in falls among those 40–64 years old compared to those in the 65 and older age group.

CHAPTER FOUR

Access to and Use of Health Services

We use data from three sources to describe access to care among adults and children in the District. First, we summarize the self-reported use of care from available survey data—the BRFSS (for adults). Second, we use information on inpatient and ED discharges from District hospitals to demonstrate the rates at which these services are used. In addition, these data allow us to identify trends in hospitalization that are sensitive to the availability and efficacy of primary care. Finally, we provide summary data from FQHCs.

4.1 Reported Use of Care Among District Adults

We use the 2011 BRFSS data to illustrate the use of preventive services among adult populations. As noted earlier, the uninsurance rate is quite low in the District (7.7 percent). Table 4.1 summarizes differences in the access to and use of preventive services among those with and without health insurance. Overall, there are significant differences in access defined by insurance. Sixty percent of those without insurance cited no regular source of care compared to only 15 percent of those with insurance. Fewer residents with insurance missed care due to cost (22 percent versus 55 percent without insurance). Further, cancer screenings (e.g., mammograms,

Table 4.1
Access to and Use of Preventive Services by Insurance Status (percentage)

Measure		Uninsured	Insured
Access (2011)	No regular source of care	60.9*	14.9*
	No routine checkup in the past year	46.9*	7.6*
	Missed care in the last 12 months because of cost	54.8*	22.4*
Preventive Care (2011)	Flu shot this year (age 65 and older)	51.2	56.9
	Pneumococcal vaccine (age 65 and older)	52.1	63.8
	HIV test (ages 18–65)	62.8*	68.4*
Cancer Screening (2010)	Mammogram within two years (women aged 50 and older)	74.2*	84.9*
	Pap smear within three years (women aged 18–64)	75.7*	91.4*
	Colonoscopy/sigmoidoscopy ever (ages 50–85)	36.7*	73.3*
	PSA or digital rectal exam (men aged 50–74)	71.0*	96.3*

* Statistically significant difference, $p < 0.05$.

pap smears, colonoscopies, and PSA tests) are more common among those with insurance compared to those without insurance.

Figure 4.1 shows medically underserved areas/populations (MUA/MUP) as defined by the U.S. Department of Health and Human Services Health Resources and Services Administration (HRSA). MUA/MUP are determined based on the index of medical underservice, which takes into consideration the ratio of primary care medical providers per 1,000 population, the infant mortality rate, the percentage of individuals living below poverty, and the percentage of persons over the age of 65. In the District, this includes census tracts around the area southeast of East Capitol and South Capitol streets, Anacostia, and the homeless population of downtown, as well as low-income populations in Brentwood, Columbia Heights, Fort Totten, and Takoma (HRSA, 2012). Figure 4.2 shows primary care health professional shortage areas (HPSAs) in the District, which are very similar to the MUA/MUP. Primary care HPSAs are defined as having a population to full-time equivalent primary care physician ratio of less than 3,500:1 but greater than 3,000:1 and having high primary care service needs and insufficient provider capacity. In the District, primary care HPSAs include several health centers: Mary's Center, Unity, Community of Hope, La Clinica del Pueblo, Whitman Walker Clinic, Elaine Ellis Center of Health, and Family and Medical Counseling Service. In addition, these HPSAs include the homeless population of downtown, as well as low-income populations in Brentwood, Columbia Heights, Fort Totten, and Takoma and census tracts southeast of East Capitol Street and around South Capitol Street (HRSA, 2012).

Figure 4.3 shows the location of several District health facilities. United Medical Center is the only hospital serving the population east of the Anacostia River. The primary care centers

Figure 4.1
Medically Underserved Areas/Populations in the District

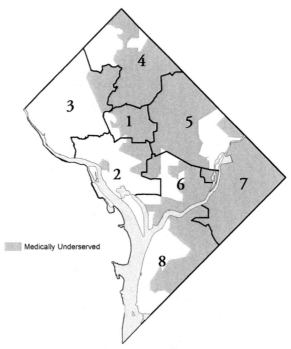

SOURCE: HRSA, 2012.
RAND *RR207-4.1*

Figure 4.2
Primary Care Health Professional Shortage Areas in the District

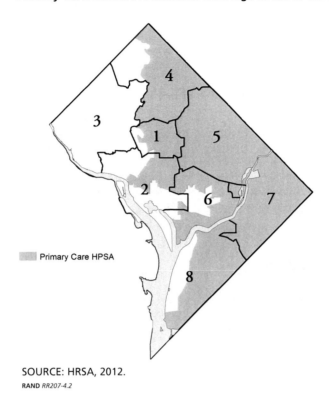

SOURCE: HRSA, 2012.
RAND *RR207-4.2*

Figure 4.3
Hospitals and Primary Care Centers in the District

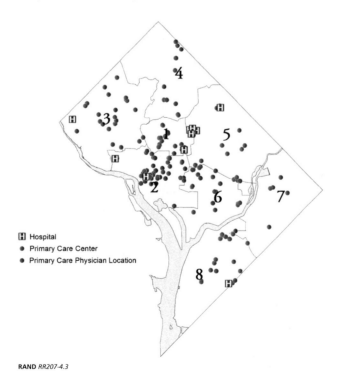

RAND *RR207-4.3*

shown include community clinics and health centers listed above. As noted, these centers are concentrated in medically underserved or primary care HPSAs. Also identified are locations of primary care physician practices, which are concentrated downtown, adjacent to hospitals, and in the northwest.

Figure 4.4 shows mental health HPSAs. To qualify as a mental health HPSA, an area or population must have a population-to-core mental health provider ratio greater than or equal to 6,000:1 and a population-to-psychiatrist ratio greater than or equal to 20,000:1, or, alternatively, a population-to-core professional ratio greater than or equal to 9,000:1 or a population-to-psychiatrist ratio greater than or equal to 30,000:1. Higher provider-to-patient ratios are often permitted in areas with high mental health needs. In the District, mental health HPSAs are present in Anacostia and also include several health centers: Mary's Center, Unity, Community of Hope, La Clinica del Pueblo, Whitman Walker Clinic, Elaine Ellis Center of Health, and Family and Medical Counseling Service (HRSA, 2012).

4.2 Inpatient and ED Discharges

We analyzed 2000–2011 (with particular focus on 2006–2011, to examine recency effects) hospital discharge data to describe rates of inpatient and ED discharges over time, where the numerator is the number of discharges among District residents and the denominator is the population of District residents.

Figure 4.4
Mental Health Professional Shortage Areas in the District

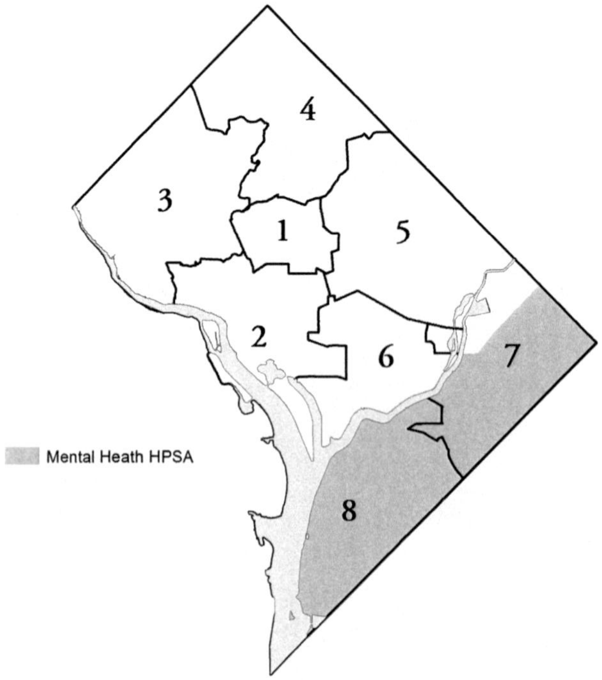

SOURCE: HRSA, 2012.
RAND *RR207-4.4*

Inpatient Discharges

Table 4.2 profiles trends over time in hospital discharge rates in the District by patient age. From 2006 to 2011, overall discharge rates for D.C. residents remained fairly steady, but between 2006 and 2011, rates among those 65 and older fell from 299 to 269 per 1,000 population and among 18–39-year-olds from 81 to 69 per 1,000 population. Since 2000, the sharpest decline in inpatient discharges (per 1,000 population) was in the 65 and older age group (Figure 4.5).

Wards 7 and 8 have reported the most inpatient discharges among youth aged 0–17 years and adults aged 18–64 years. Ward 5 has the highest rate of discharges among those older than 65 years, though that rate has steadily declined over the past ten years (Figure 4.6).

The volume of inpatient discharges does differ by hospital. Not surprisingly, Children's National Medical Center experiences the greatest number of discharges in the 0–17 age group; George Washington University Hospital reports the most in the 65 and older age group; and Washington Hospital Center reports the most in the adult population between 18 and 64 years old (Figure 4.7).

ED Discharges

Table 4.3 profiles ED utilization rates among District residents by age over the 2006–2011 period. Discharge rates were steady among those aged 0–17 through 2009 and then increased substantially in 2010 and 2011(see also Figure 4.8).

Rates were general steady for all other age groups. Please note, however, that we do not include United Medical Center data in this analysis due to data unavailability at the time of the study, thus declines in the rates among the adult population may be somewhat exaggerated. In total, ED discharges increased 8 percent between 2006 and 2011.

As with inpatient discharges, the highest rate of ED discharges among youth (0–17 years old) and adults (18–64 years old) was in Wards 7 and 8. ED discharges were highest among those 65 and older in Ward 5 (Figure 4.9). In contrast to inpatient discharge rates, however, Washington Hospital Center noted the highest number of discharges among all adults, including those 65 years and older (Figure 4.10).

4.3 Reasons for Inpatient and ED Discharges

We examined the top conditions across all hospitals for inpatient and ED discharges (Tables 4.4 and 4.5). For inpatient discharges, the top conditions are diseases of the heart, complica-

Table 4.2
Inpatient Admissions Among District Residents per 1,000 Population (2006–2011)

Age	2006	2007	2008	2009	2010	2011
0–17	43	39	43	43	49	46
18–39	81	79	80	79	69	69
40–64	153	147	149	150	151	151
65 and older	299	283	290	282	281	269
All	121	116	119	118	114	112

SOURCE: Authors' analyses of DCHA data.

Figure 4.5
Total D.C. Inpatient Discharges per 1,000 Population by Age

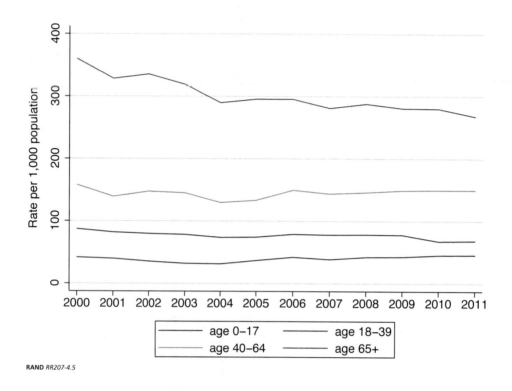

RAND *RR207-4.5*

Figure 4.6
Inpatient Discharges per 1,000 Population by Ward and Age

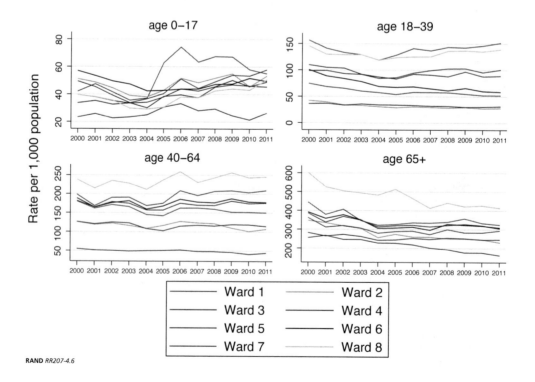

RAND *RR207-4.6*

Figure 4.7
Total Inpatient Discharges by Hospital and Age

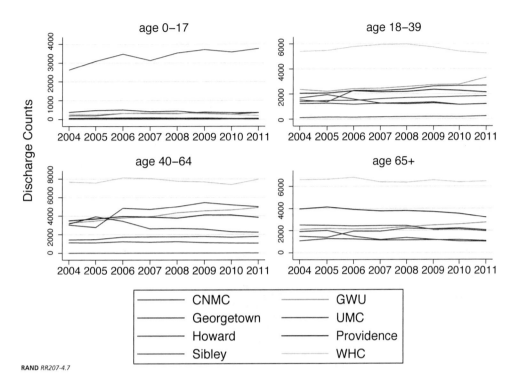

RAND *RR207-4.7*

tions related to injury and poisoning, or pregnancy. For ED discharges, respiratory infections and contusions are the second and third most cited, respectively, though conditions without a clear diagnosis top the list. For more detail about how these common conditions vary by year, see Appendix A.

Trends by Hospital

Top conditions for inpatient discharges vary by hospital. For example, the top condition for United Medical Center in 2011 was schizophrenia, followed by diseases of the heart. For Children's National Medical Center, respiratory infections, epilepsy, and asthma top the list in that

Table 4.3
ED Discharges Among District Residents per 1,000 Population (2006–2011)

Age	2006	2007	2008	2009	2010	2011
0–17	410	420	438	465	513	640
18–39	342	335	348	313	299	309
40–64	416	420	440	393	433	444
65 and older	307	314	326	299	326	333
All	374	376	391	365	377	408

SOURCE: Authors' analyses of DCHA data.

Figure 4.8
Total D.C. ED Discharges per 1,000 Population by Age

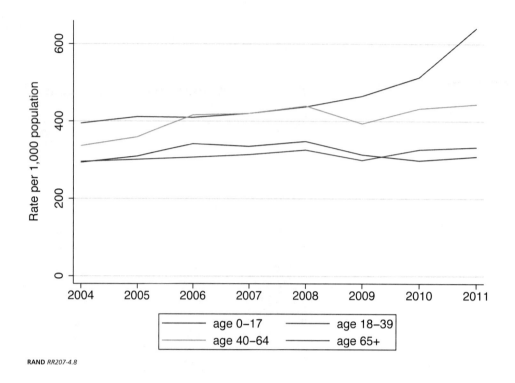

Figure 4.9
Total ED Discharges per 1,000 Population by Age and Ward

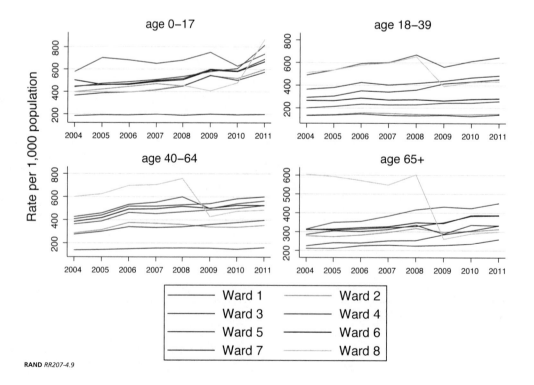

Figure 4.10
Total ED Discharges by Hospital and Age

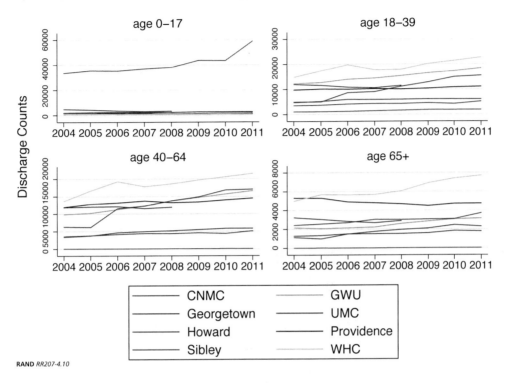

RAND RR207-4.10

order. For George Washington University Hospital, diseases of the heart and urinary issues are the top two conditions. Howard University Hospital and Providence Hospital also note diseases of the heart as the top conditions, and Sibley indicates its top condition for inpatient discharges is complications due to pregnancy.

Table 4.4
Most Frequent Primary Conditions for Inpatient Discharges from District Hospitals (2011)

Primary Condition (using Condition Classification System)	Rank (based on total discharges)
[07.02] Diseases of the heart	1
[16.10] Complications related to injury and poisoning	2
[11.03] Complications mainly related to pregnancy	3
[10.01] Diseases of the urinary system	4
[07.03] Cerebrovascular disease	5
[11.04] Indications for care in pregnancy; labor; and delivery	6
[05.08] Mood disorders	7
[09.06] Lower gastrointestinal disorders	8
[11.06] Other complications of birth; puerperium affecting management of mother	9
[16.02] Fractures	10

Table 4.5
Most Frequent Primary Conditions for ED Discharges from District Hospitals (2011)

Primary Condition (using Condition Classification System)	Rank (based on total discharges)
[17.01] Symptoms; signs; and ill-defined conditions	1
[08.01] Respiratory infections	2
[16.08] Superficial injury; contusion	3
[16.07] Sprains and strains	4
[16.06] Open wounds	5
[07.02] Diseases of the heart	6
[06.08] Ear conditions	7
[13.03] Spondylosis; intervertebral disc disorders; other back problems	8
[10.01] Diseases of the urinary system	9
[16.12] Other injuries and conditions due to external causes	10

For ED discharges, George Washington University, Providence, and Sibley Hospitals most frequently diagnose using the general symptoms and ill-defined conditions code. Respiratory infections top the list at Children's National Medical Center for ED discharges. Howard University Hospital's top condition is sprains and associated injuries. Note that United Medical Center's ED data are not available.

4.4 Ambulatory Care Sensitive Inpatient and ED Discharges

We use 2000–2011 DCHA data to describe trends in hospitalizations sensitive to the availability and effectiveness of outpatient services, such as primary and specialty care. These are referred to as ambulatory care sensitive (ACS) hospitalizations and are used as a proxy of the availability and use of primary and preventive health services. Often, the ACS is used to identify communities where need is high yet health service availability is low or health service use is inappropriate.

Figures 4.11–4.17 show trends over time in ACS hospitalizations by age group (0–17, 18–39, 40–64, 65 and over) and patient residence (ward), as well as by hospital. ACS rates are calculated for the District by dividing the number of ACS discharges for a particular age group by the size of the population in that age group over time from 2000 to 2011. We calculated ACS rates for inpatient and ED discharges.

The trends shown in the figures are as follows:

- ACS inpatient discharges have sharply declined among those 65 and older but held steady across all other age groups.
- ACS inpatient discharges are highest among those 0–17 years old, 18–39 years old, and 40–64 years old in Wards 7 and 8; but are highest in Ward 5 among those 65 and older, though that rate has sharply declined.
- ACS inpatient discharges are more common (in terms of total count) among those in the 18 and older age group served by Washington Hospital Center. The total number of dis-

charges among those 0–17 years old is greatest among those served by Children's National Medical Center; while this is not surprising, what is notable is the sharp increase in the total discharges after 2006. As a percentage of overall discharges, Children's National Medical Center experiences the most ACS inpatient discharges, followed by United Medical Center and Howard University Hospital (see Figure 4.14).

- ACS ED discharges are greatest among those 0–17 years old, with a sharp increase in 2010 and 2011. This increase appears to have been driven by ED discharges in Ward 8, followed by Ward 7.
- Overall, ACS ED discharges are more prevalent among adults served by Washington Hospital Center, followed by George Washington University Hospital and Providence Hospital.

4.5 Inpatient and ED Discharge Rates by Diagnosis

We looked at trends over time in specific diagnoses associated with ACS discharges for children and adults (e.g., asthma, diabetes, sepsis, and cellulitis). In addition, we explored some trends in diagnoses that showed increasing patterns over the last several years (e.g., alcohol-related ED discharges).

Figure 4.11
ACS Inpatient Discharges per 1,000 Population by Age (all D.C.)

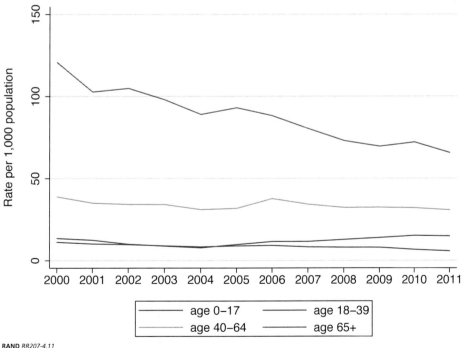

RAND RR207-4.11

Figure 4.12
ACS Inpatient Discharges per 1,000 Population in the District by Age and Ward

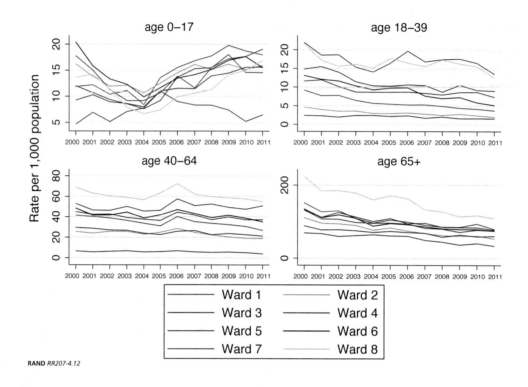

RAND *RR207-4.12*

Figure 4.13
ACS Inpatient Discharges in the District by Hospital and Age

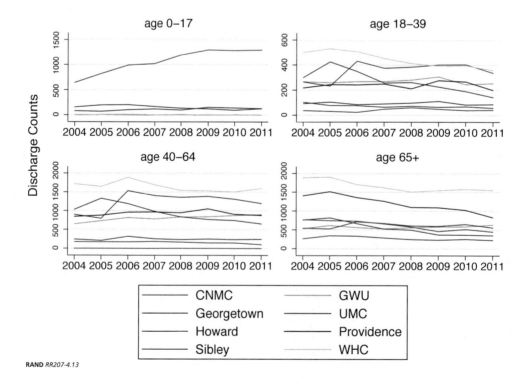

RAND *RR207-4.13*

Figure 4.14
ACS Inpatient Discharges as a Percentage of Total Hospital Discharges in the District (2011)

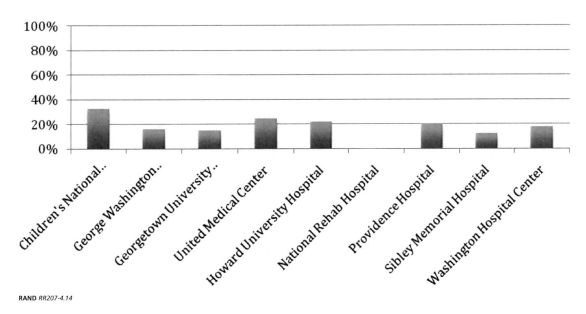

Figure 4.15
ACS ED Discharges per 1,000 Population in the District by Age

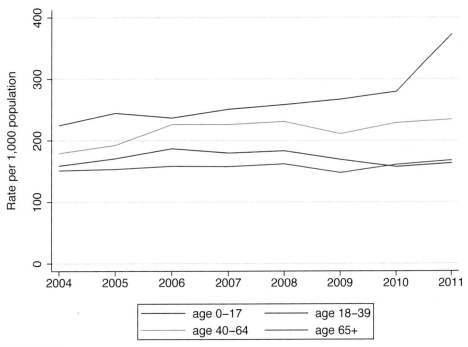

Figure 4.16
ACS ED Discharges per 1,000 Population in the District by Age and Ward

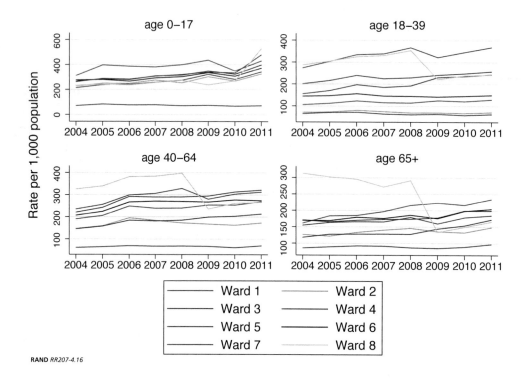

RAND RR207-4.16

Figure 4.17
ACS ED Discharges in the District by Hospital and Age

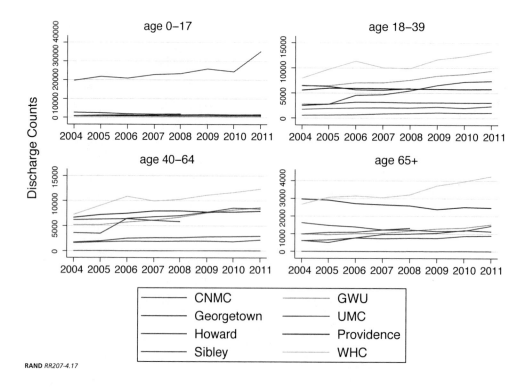

RAND RR207-4.17

For children, asthma and bacterial infections comprise a large percentage of ACS inpatient rates (see Figure 4.18). For adults, the main drivers for inpatient discharges are generally sepsis, coronary atherosclerosis (though that is declining), and congestive heart failure. For ED discharges, key diagnoses are asthma, conditions related to alcohol, and back pain. We detail the trends for each diagnosis below.

Asthma

Asthma is a key condition in calculating ACS hospitalizations. For inpatient discharges, asthma rates among those 0–17 years old experienced some decline in 2004 but have sharply increased since that point (reaching nearly 4.5 per 1,000 population in 2011) (Figure 4.19). These rates are highest among 0–17-year-olds in Wards 7 and 8, followed by 40–64-year-olds in the same wards (Figure 4.20).

Looking at asthma-related ED discharges, rates have also significantly increased among 0–17 year olds, particularly after 2010 (Figure 4.21), and show the same patterns by ward (Figure 4.22). Because we calculated asthma-related visits using the population as a numerator, the number may not accurately reflect hospitalization by asthma rate. There is some evidence that rates of asthma have increased in the District, in which case the rise in asthma hospitalization and ED rates may actually be less steep than reported in our report, though those analyses are currently unpublished.

Figure 4.18
ACS Inpatient Discharges by Condition in the District for 0–17-Year-Olds

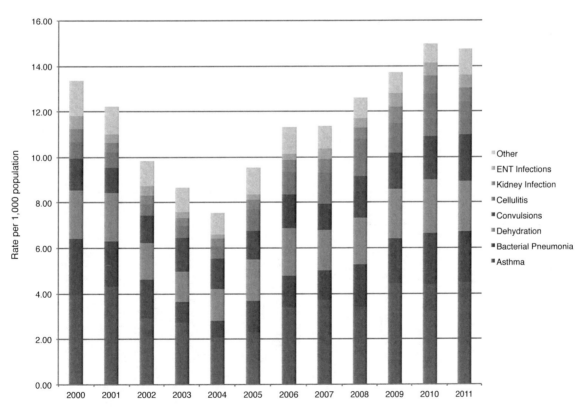

Figure 4.19
Asthma Inpatient Discharges per 1,000 Population in the District by Age

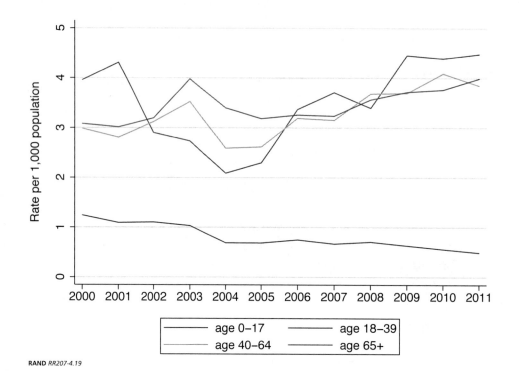

Figure 4.20
Asthma Inpatient Discharges per 1,000 Population in the District by Ward and Age

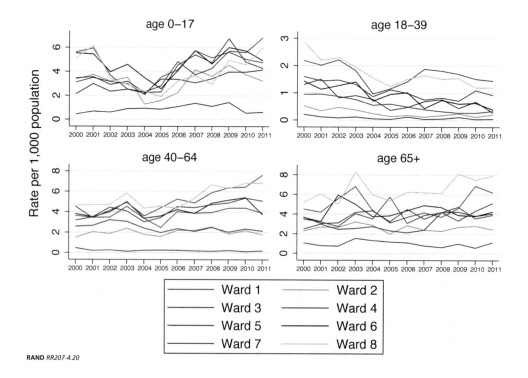

Figure 4.21
Asthma ED Discharges per 1,000 Population in the District by Age

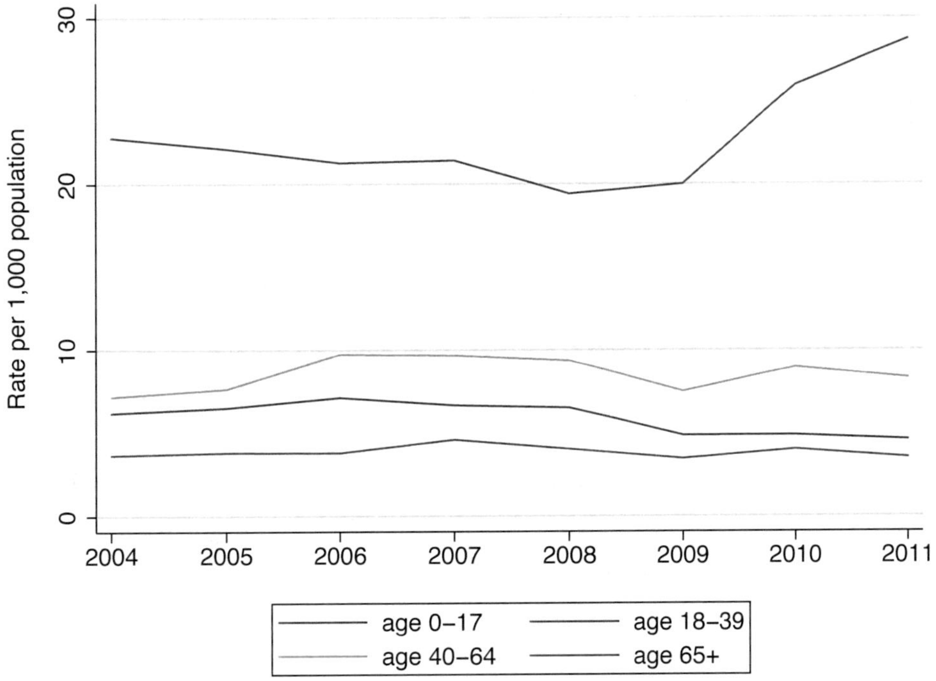

RAND *RR207-4.21*

Diabetes

Diabetes is also a key condition for calculating ACS hospitalizations, particularly inpatient discharges. Inpatient discharges for diabetes have declined among the older age groups (40–65 years and older) but have held steady among younger age groups (Figure 4.23). By ward, there is a lot of variability in inpatient discharges, particularly among 0–17-year-olds in Wards 7 and 8, where there have been sharp increases and decreases since 2006. Otherwise, the rates have held steady, with some decline in discharges in Ward 5 among those 65 and older (Figure 4.24).

Sepsis and Cellulitis

Both sepsis (i.e., infection) and cellulitis (a skin infection) are considered avoidable conditions (if prevented) that often require inpatient discharges. There has not been much improvement in the rates of these diagnoses in the District over the last decade. Sepsis-related discharges are still high among those 65 years and older (Figure 4.25) and most common among those in Ward 5. The rate of cellulitis is also fairly high and generally steady among all age groups, with some increase since 2008 among those 0–17 years old (Figure 4.26).

Heart Disease

One of the most notable trends over the last few years is a sharp decline in heart disease–related discharges, particularly those related to coronary atherosclerosis (Figure 4.27).

This downward slope is primarily driven by declines in discharges among those 65 and older across all wards (Figure 4.28). Rates of congestive heart failure and acute myocardial

Figure 4.22
Asthma ED Discharges per 1,000 Population in the District by Ward and Age

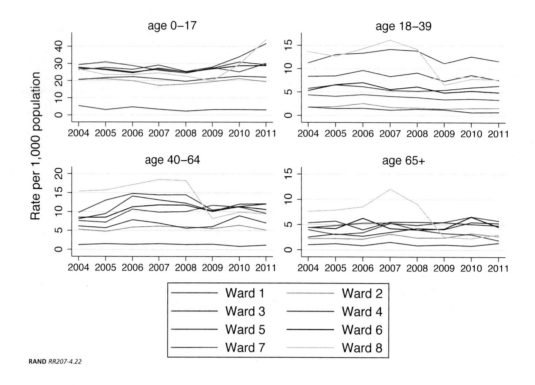

RAND *RR207-4.22*

Figure 4.23
Diabetes Inpatient Discharges per 1,000 Population in the District by Age

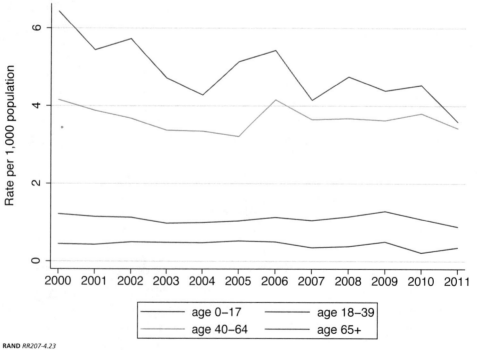

RAND *RR207-4.23*

Figure 4.24
Diabetes Inpatient Discharges per 1,000 Population by Ward and Age

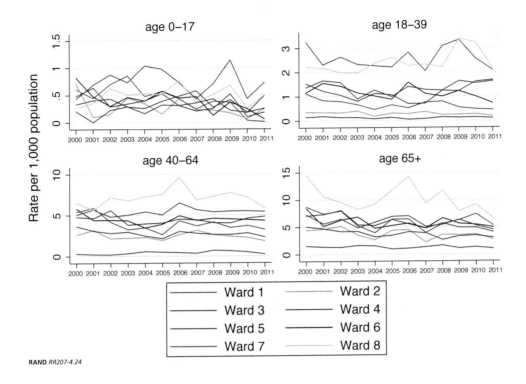

Figure 4.25
Sepsis-Related Inpatient Discharges per 1,000 Population in the District by Age

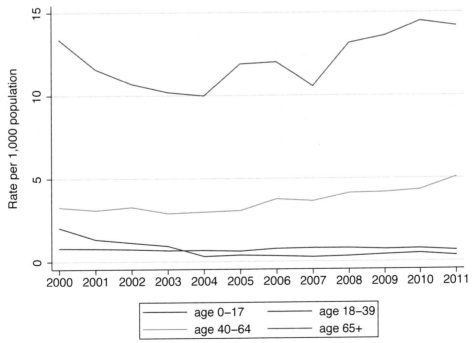

Figure 4.26
Cellulitis-Related Inpatient Discharges per 1,000 Population in the District by Age

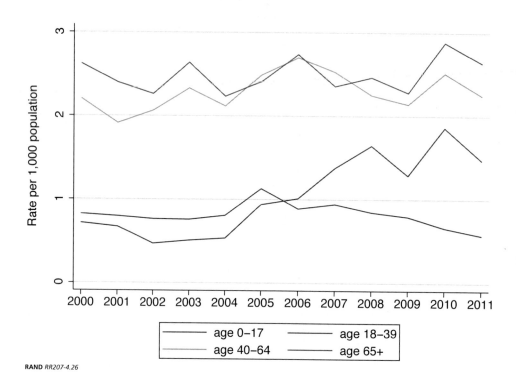

infarctions (i.e., heart attack) have also declined in this age group and across all wards, though not as sharply as the rate of atherosclerosis. Reasons for this are unclear but could include improved service use in outpatient sectors and/or the increased use of medication.

Stress-Related Diagnoses

A key trend in ED discharges over the past few years has been in the area of "stress-related discharges," namely headaches, migraines, and back pain among adults. We term these conditions *stress-related* because they tend to be exacerbated by stress. The rate of back pain ED discharges has sharply increased, especially among those 40–64 years old (Figure 4.29). This increase appears to be greatest in this age group among those in Wards 5, 6, and 7. These conditions are less common in Wards 2 and 3 (Figure 4.30). George Washington University Hospital, Washington Hospital Center, Providence Hospital, and Howard University Hospital report the most back pain ED discharges.

Similarly, headache and migraine discharge have been increasing since 2009 among 40–64-year-olds, particularly in Wards 5 and 7 (Figure 4.31). The same hospital patterns persist for these conditions as for back pain.

Alcohol-Related Discharges

Concurrently, alcohol-related ED discharges increased among 40–64-years-olds from 15 per 1,000 population in 2009 to 19 per 1,000 population in 2011. For these discharges, the sharpest increases are among 18–39-year-olds living in Ward 1 and 40–64-year-olds living in Wards 1 and 5 (Figure 4.32). Howard University Hospital reports the most discharges among 18–64-year-olds related to alcohol.

Figure 4.27
Inpatient Discharges in the District Due to Heart Disease

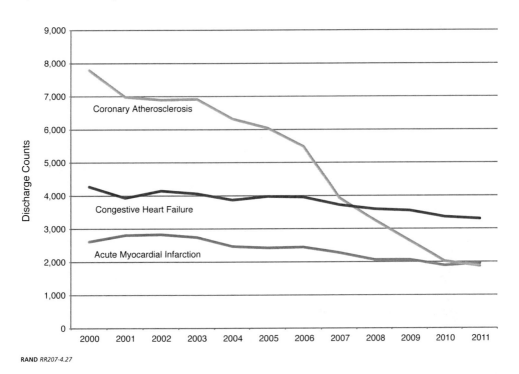

RAND *RR207-4.27*

Figure 4.28
Coronary Atherosclerosis Inpatient Discharges per 1,000 Population in the District by Age

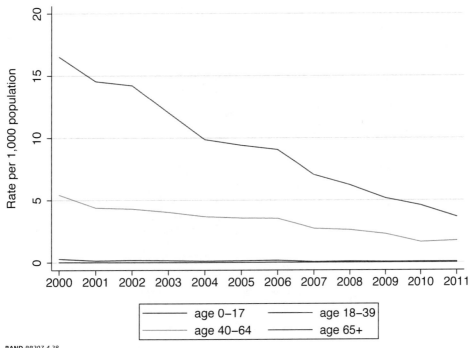

RAND *RR207-4.28*

Figure 4.29
Back Pain ED Discharges per 1,000 Population by Age

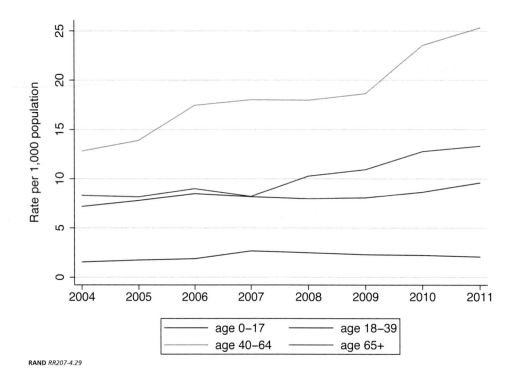

RAND *RR207-4.29*

Figure 4.30
Back Pain ED Discharges per 1,000 Population in the District by Ward and Age

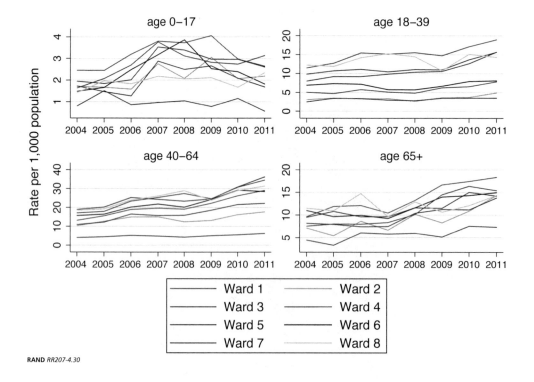

RAND *RR207-4.30*

Figure 4.31
Headache- and Migraine-Related ED Discharges per 1,000 Population in the District by Ward and Age

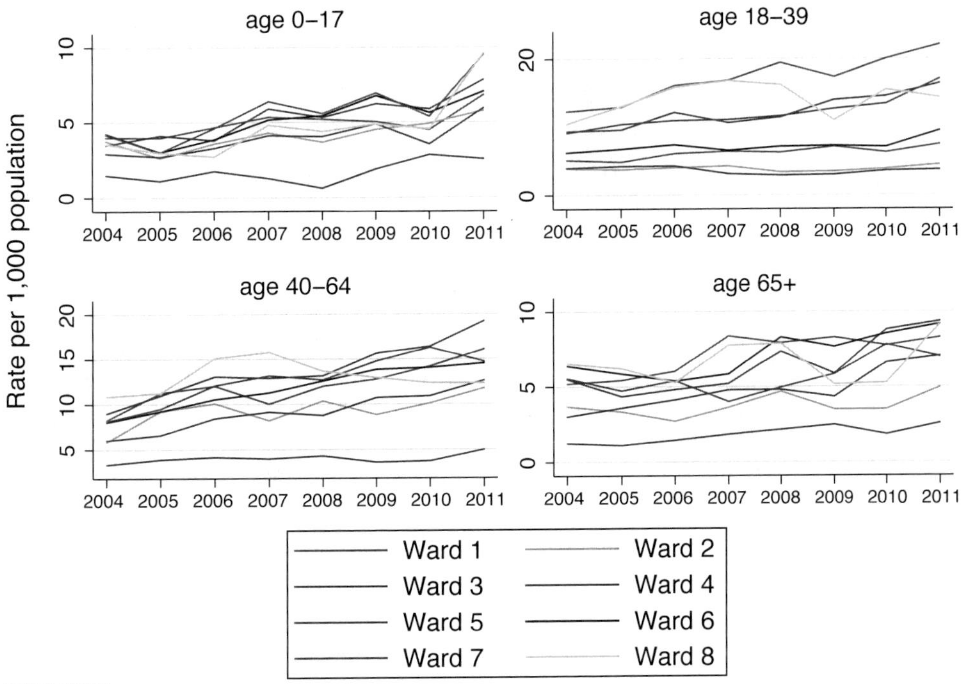

RAND RR207-4.31

4.6 Federally Qualified Health Centers

Unity Health Care, Community of Hope, La Clinica del Pueblo, and Mary's Center comprise the four District grantees designated as FQHCs and captured in the national Uniform Data System (UDS) as of the time of this study. In 2011, there were a total of 122,891 patients served by these clinics, with 45 percent of these patients being male and 55 percent female. Approximately 60 percent of the population lived 100 percent or more below the federal poverty level, 55 percent used Medicaid, and less than 4 percent had private insurance.

Table 4.4 details the total number of patients with key primary diagnoses, as well as the total number of visits. Approximately 9 percent of patients had a primary diagnosis of overweight or obesity, 7 percent had asthma, and 7 percent had diabetes. Given the obesity rates in the city generally, this may be an underestimate of absolute need. Rather, this may only indicate complications from obesity for which obesity is then listed as a primary diagnosis.

Among the patients visiting these clinics (Figure 4.33), those who visit Unity and La Clinica are more often seen for hypertension, asthma patients make up a larger percentage of clients at Unity compared to the other clinics, and La Clinica sees the largest percentage of those with HIV as their primary diagnosis.

4.7 Summary

In this section, we briefly summarize key findings from our health service use analysis.

Figure 4.32
Alcohol-Related ED Discharges per 1,000 Population in the District by Ward and Age

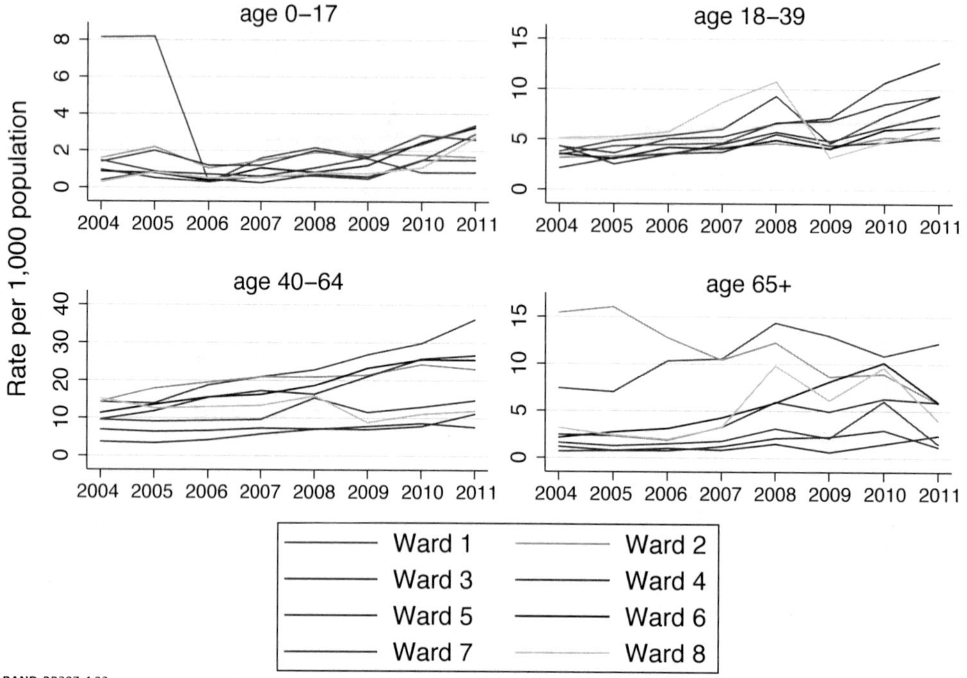

RAND RR207-4.32

Access to and Use of Preventive Services

The uninsurance rate is low in the District (7.7 percent). Sixty percent of those without insurance cited no regular source of care compared to only 15 percent with insurance. Fewer residents with insurance missed care due to cost. Cancer screening (e.g., mammograms, pap smears, colonoscopies, and PSA tests) is more common among those with insurance compared to those without insurance.

Table 4.6
Total Number of Visits and Patients Among District FQHCs by Primary Diagnosis

Diagnosis	Number of Visits	Number of Patients
Diabetes	31,908	8,627
Asthma	22,294	8,443
Overweight and obesity	17,151	10,661
HIV	16,286	2,943
Depression and other mood disorders	11,350	3,037
Other substance use disorders	7,995	4,297
Heart disease	7,145	2,327
Tobacco use disorders	5,570	3,785

SOURCE: UDS data, 2011.

Figure 4.33
District FQHC Patients with Selected Primary Diagnoses* (2011)

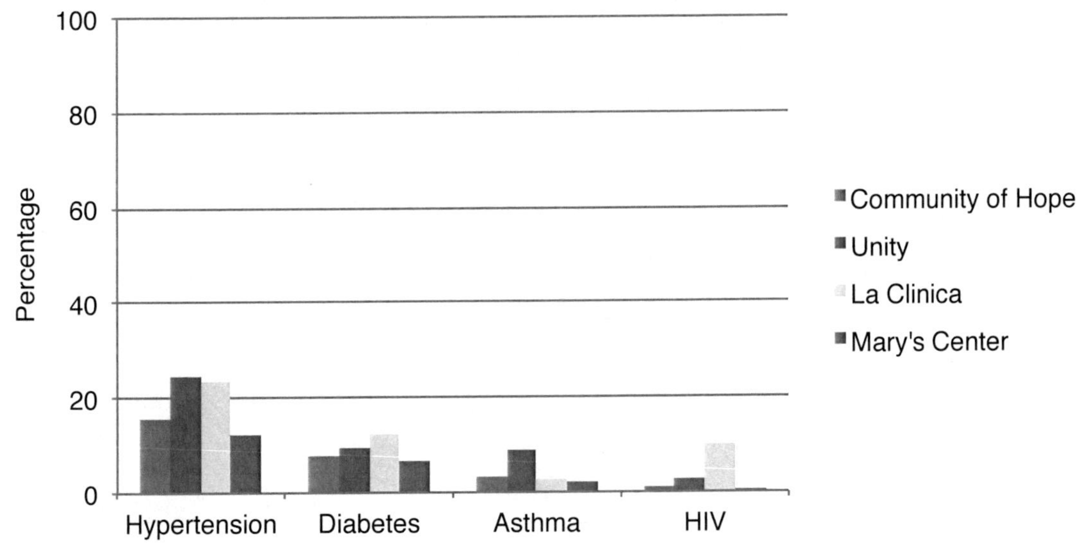

*As a percentage of each clinic's total patients.
RAND RR207-4.33

Inpatient and ED Discharges

From 2006 to 2011, overall inpatient discharge rates for D.C. residents remained fairly steady, although between 2006 and 2011 rates among those 65 and older fell from 299 to 269 per 1,000 population. For ED discharges, rates were also generally steady. However, discharge rates were steady among those 0–17 years old thorough 2009 and then increased substantially in 2010 and 2011. The top reasons for inpatient discharges are diseases of the heart, complications related to injury and poisoning, or pregnancy. For ED discharges, respiratory infections and contusions are frequently cited, though conditions without a clear diagnosis were the most common.

ACS Inpatient and ED Discharges

ACS inpatient discharges sharply declined among those 65 years and older but have held steady across all other age groups. ACS ED discharges are greatest among those 0–17 years old, with a sharp increase in 2010 and 2011. This increase appears to be driven predominantly by ED discharges in Ward 8, followed by those in Ward 7. Some key patterns in discharges by age and condition are as follows:

- For inpatient and ED discharges, asthma rates among those 0–17 years old declined some in 2004 but have sharply increased since that point.
- Sepsis-related discharges are still high among those 65 years and older and most common among those in Ward 5. The rate of cellulitis is also fairly high and generally steady among all age groups, with some increase since 2008 among those 0–17 years old.
- One of the most notable trends over the last few years is a sharp decline in heart disease–related discharges, particularly due to coronary atherosclerosis.

- A key trend in ED discharges in the past few years has been in the area of "stress-related discharges," namely headaches, migraines, and back pain. The rate of back pain ED discharges has sharply increased, especially among those 40–64 years old, with the greatest increases among this age group occurring in Wards 5, 6, and 7.

CHAPTER FIVE

Stakeholder Perspectives

To elucidate findings from our administrative and survey data analysis, we conducted focus groups with key stakeholders who are advocates or providers of health and social services. We did not include community residents, as those groups were surveyed by DOH, and this report focused on recommendations that could be implemented by organizations (hence the inclusion of organization leaders). The primary objectives of these focus groups were:

- to identify priority health and health care issues, as well as critical service needs to which stakeholders feel greater investment should be targeted
- to understand how social determinants impact health and health service use in the city
- to understand the barriers to addressing health and related social factors
- to identify recommendations for the DCHCC to improve health and social services in the city
- to identify additional data that health and social service stakeholders would find beneficial in the DC Health Matters portal.

In the sections that follow, we describe our methodology and present key findings from our focus groups.

5.1 Methods

We conducted four focus groups from October to November 2012 with a total of 30 participants. Two of the focus groups focused on health and health service issues. Two of the focus groups focused on social determinants and related social service issues that impact health. The focus group participants were recruited from health, social service, and advocacy agencies that catered to individual wards, as well as the broader District community. Final participants included hospital patient advocates, case managers, Department of Health officials, and community-based health and social services stakeholders. We queried stakeholders about a number of major issues, including what they viewed as priority health and social services needs for the city in general, the particular needs that were relevant to the populations they served, and their specific recommendations for concrete steps that could be implemented to improve overall health and social service for residents, with a specific focus on the steps that DCHCC members should take. For a complete focus group protocol, please see Appendix B of this report.

The next sections present the major themes we identified in our focus groups using summary points and, in some cases, illustrative quotes from participants. The themes are ordered first by issues that relate to health and health services (e.g., behavioral health, specialty services), then issues related to social services and other determinants of health (e.g., case management). Table 5.1 summarizes our findings and recommendations.

5.2 Behavioral Health

Behavioral health remains a significant problem for D.C. residents, particularly those with Medicaid and those who do not speak English. Focus group participants noted that the capacity for psychiatric services in the District is limited. More psychiatrists and psychologists are needed, particularly to serve the Medicaid population. There are limited referral options for outpatient behavioral health services, and there are extended waiting times for evaluation. Further, participants raised concerns that some persons may not know about their diagnosis or available treatment options. There are also few skilled nursing beds available to treat per-

Table 5.1
Key Findings and Recommendations from Focus Groups

	Findings	Recommendations
Behavioral Health	• Behavioral health services are limited for persons with Medicaid, as well as for persons for whom English is not a primary language. • Few transitional services exist for persons with behavioral health needs. • Treatment options for comorbid medical conditions associated with behavioral health issues are limited.	• More support services are needed for persons with behavioral health issues particularly for persons with Medicaid and for whom English is not a primary language. • More supportive services are needed to support independent living among persons with behavioral health needs. • More skilled nursing beds are needed for persons with behavioral health needs.
Obesity and Nutrition	• There is a shortage of family targeted interventions that address obesity and promote healthy eating.	• Family-based programs targeting obesity are needed, such as healthy shopping and family-oriented education programs.
Preventive Health Services	• Hospitals focus mainly on treatment services instead of preventive health services. • There is a lack of coordination between health and social service agencies to work in concert to provide preventive services.	• Programs that support healthy behaviors are needed. • Hospitals should engage social service organizations in developing and promoting preventive health programs.
Specialty Services	• Lack of specialists, especially in Wards 7 and 8, leads to delays between diagnosis and treatment for certain conditions, particularly oncology care and pain management services.	• Provider incentives and partnerships, such as loan repayment programs and specialists in community based health organizations as part of their training experience, may help provide needed specialty services in areas where there are shortages.

Table 5.1—Continued

	Findings	Recommendations
Eldercare and End-of-Life Services	• Expanded services for the elderly are needed to help support family members who care for them in the community. • Residents are not well informed about hospice and end-of-life care services.	• More resources to help families who care for the elderly are needed, including expanded case management services.
Disability Services	• Adequate services for persons with disabilities are lacking in the city. • Health care providers are not comfortable treating persons with disabilities.	• Programs should provide health and social services for persons with disabilities at all life stages. • Providers should be better educated to address the unique health care needs of persons with disabilities.
Information Technology	• Lack of linkage of information technology systems across health care organizations results in duplicative services.	• There is a need for linkage of medical records across hospitals and outpatient clinics similar to that of the previously existing DC Regional Health Information System (RHIO).
Case Management	• Hospitals and clinics do not offer convenient hours or co-located services • There is little linkage of case management services across hospital sites to provide continuity of care for residents who use services at multiple sites; there is also little linkage of residents to medical homes at discharge. • Few resources exist to link children with chronic health needs from pediatric to adult providers as they transition into adulthood.	• Greater case management services are needed to link residents across medical services across hospitals and with medical homes in the community. • Patient navigation should be expanded to help direct residents to services across a number of chronic diseases and for children as they transition into adulthood.
Social Determinants and Social Services	• Health is viewed as a lower priority among residents who are faced with poverty and unemployment. • Immigrants are uncomfortable using services due to fear of documentation requirements. • Cultural competency is lacking among health care providers. • Language services can be difficult to provide due to prohibitive costs. • Wards 7 and 8 have few health and social services, and residents are often not well informed about those services that do exist. • There is inadequate housing support for homeless individuals, particularly those with special needs. • Interventions often are not tailored to address persons with varying literacy levels. • Residents have little trust in District hospitals.	• The medical community needs better awareness of social determinants that impact health. • Cultural competency training is needed for providers to help address the needs of residents from diverse backgrounds. • Health care organizations must form partnerships with social organizations and build upon the existing social capital within a community. • Hospitals and FQHCs should go into the community to educate residents about health resources. • A centralized resource list of available community based health and social services is needed. • Expanded housing options for the homeless are needed. • Messages must be tailored to address residents of all literacy levels.

sons with behavioral health needs who require more intensive long-term management of other comorbid medical conditions, such as diabetes or hypertension.

One participant noted:

> Access to mental health services is not good. The crisis line is always backed up and there are [few] psychiatrists.

Many of the patient advocates noted that persons with mental illness use hospital EDs due to a lack of adequate social service support in the community. In addition, stigma associated with mental health leads to lower motivation to use community-based services. Participants also cited a lack of services targeted toward Spanish-speaking individuals and persons with limited English-speaking ability. Such limitations augment an already large need for mental health services in the District. In particular, there are limited detoxification centers located in the community and accessible to persons from diverse patient backgrounds, including non-English-speaking individuals. According to one participant:

> There are only three facilities in the city that provide substance abuse [counseling] in Spanish and no detox.

Participants noted a lack of transitional services, including housing and job training, that allow persons with behavioral health needs to function more independently in the community. Again, these services are particularly limited for persons with limited English-speaking capacity.

5.3 Obesity and Nutrition

Participants articulated concerns that interventions targeting obesity are limited for residents in the District. In particular, few programs that focus on behavioral change for the entire family are available. Resources to promote good nutrition are limited, particularly in Wards 7 and 8. Although there has been greater focus on providing healthy options in neighborhoods, such as through community-based corner stores, residents are not often aware of these alternatives. In addition, participants raised concerns that residents are not aware of healthy exercise options available in their community, such as the location of parks, bike lanes, or Capital Bikshare sites.

5.4 Preventive Health Services

Participants noted that most hospitals and clinics did not place enough emphasis on preventive health, which could help decrease long-term, high-cost treatments. Obesity and nutrition were examples given of areas where prevention efforts are particularly limited. This was noted by both hospital-based and community-based providers, including those at Medicaid managed care plans. Participants believed many insurance plans, particularly managed care plans, did not adequately educate or remind residents about the need for preventive tests, such as mammograms or prostate screening.

Hospitals should advocate for policies that are pro-health, not necessarily pro-medicine ... [insurance] should reimburse for nutrition education and physical activity education, not just bariatric surgery.

5.5 Specialty Services

Participants identified problems with obtaining specialty care in the District, especially for persons who live in Wards 7 and 8. Oncology and pain management services were identified as being particularly problematic. Case managers and patient advocates cited pain management as an issue leading to frequent ED use.

Few oncologists practice in Wards 7 and 8. Also, it is particularly difficult for persons to navigate the system to access oncology services both in the community and at various hospitals. Because of the limited number of specialists available, particularly for oncology, participants noted that residents, particularly those living in Wards 7 and 8, often have to wait for prolonged periods following diagnosis to obtain needed medical care. Poor reimbursement and a lack of motivation for doctors to donate charity care were cited as factors contributing to the shortage of specialists in underserved areas of the city.

Due to limited outpatient pain management services in certain neighborhoods, participants noted that residents sometimes use the ED to help meet their treatment needs. When available, pain management is often limited or medications are provided in a restricted capacity that does not adequately address the medication needs of affected individuals.

5.6 Eldercare and End-of-Life Services

Participants recommended expanded services for the elderly to help support the family members who care for them in the community. Many elderly in the District are cared for at home by family members who often have limited support. Patient navigators noted that there are limited community-based resources available to such family caregivers, and when services exist, they are not well known. Participants also noted a lack of mental health services targeted to the elderly. In particular, there are a limited number of skilled nursing facility beds for the elderly with mental health needs.

Additionally, participants explained that residents are not well informed about hospice and end-of-life care services. Community-based hospice services are often limited and residents do not have a clear understanding of how to use such services. One participant commented:

With the terminally ill, there are no discussions about advance directives, no thought of hospice, and no advanced care planning.

5.7 Disability Services

The disabled population is not extensively addressed in many health and social service interventions, yet this population is in need and represents a growing segment of the city. Participants noted that few services were available to this population. Because the disabled are living longer, they face a number of comorbid medical conditions, including dementia, and they often have concurrent social service needs. Participants explained that families who care for such individuals are not well equipped, given the lack of appropriate case management and the lack of connections to community-based support services. In addition, services do not adequately address persons throughout all stages of the life continuum. One participant noted that neighboring jurisdictions, such as Virginia and Maryland, have more services directed at the coordination of care for persons with disabilities at birth than does the District.

In addition, some participants felt that providers are often uncomfortable treating persons with disabilities and that this may result in the failure to provide comprehensive treatment and coordination of care. This discomfort may be due to a lack of appropriate training and education in dealing with the disabled population.

5.8 Information Technology

A few participants also shared concerns that information exchange between hospitals and clinics is limited since there is no technology linking hospital databases. Participants noted the benefits the D.C. Regional Health Information Organization (RHIO) provided during its short-lived existence. RHIO allowed hospitals and some clinics to have access to medical records across sites, which participants felt reduced unnecessary tests and duplicative services.

5.9 Case Management and Care Coordination

Participants cited inconvenient hours and locations of providers and the lack of colocated services as being particularly challenging. These challenge are amplified for persons with Medicaid or who have special social service needs. Work schedules often prevent residents from accessing outpatient services during operating hours, especially when multiple tests are required that cannot be obtained all in the same day. Participants also discussed how frequent health care users often use multiple hospitals, resulting in duplicative services, and cited poor linkage across medical sites, which makes it difficult for case managers to work in concert across hospitals to coordinate care. Case managers noted that there is often a lack of access to up-to-date information for residents on discharge to ensure continuity of care and long-term disease management. Further, participants shared that there are few resources available to help children with chronic health needs transition into adulthood. Case managers who care for pediatric populations often do not have established relationships with case managers who care for adult populations, making this transition more difficult.

5.10 Social Determinants and Associated Social Services

We also asked participants about a number of social determinants that affect health, as well as services that could help address such determinants. Participants cited a number of determinants, including poverty, unemployment, language and immigration status, homelessness, and illiteracy.

Participants felt that high poverty and unemployment rates made health services less effective. When individuals have to focus on such problems as poverty and unemployment, they are likely to place lower priority on receiving health services. Without first addressing these underlying social issues and how to remedy them, it would be hard to address health issues. As one participant explained:

> Health is not my number one priority when I am unemployed.

Participants also noted that undocumented immigrants can face many barriers that discourage their use of health and social services. Often immigrants with health needs in D.C. are less likely to use services because they fear repercussions due to their legal status. Programs that require extensive paperwork and documentation may discourage immigrants from using services that can provide great benefit. Additionally, participants raised concerns that inadequate cultural competency restricts social and health service agencies' ability to deal with residents from diverse racial and ethnic backgrounds. Members of the District's Latino population, for example, come from a diverse spectrum of backgrounds, which health and social service providers often may not understand. Participants expressed concern that social service agencies are mandated to provide access to translation services but often do not have adequate resources to meet this expensive provision. As one participant stated:

> Not all Latinos are the same. People that work with Latinos in D.C. need background info on where most of [them] come from. . . . They might know how to speak Spanish, but they don't understand the context of the Latino community.

Participants also noted the homeless population as being particularly underserved in terms of health and social services. Many services, such as the hypothermia van, are inconvenient (for example, one patient advocate noted that to be picked up by the hypothermia van, the client had to be standing outside in the cold). Often the homeless use hospitals for social services because of inadequate community-based resources for this population. As one participant stated:

> The homeless population will go to every hospital for food. We can't put them where they need [to go]. . . . We need more skilled places for [the] homeless.

In addition, there are few affordable housing options for the homeless. There is a lack of programs, in particular, that focus on long-term placement rather than filling a temporary need. Participants stated that there was a limited capacity of specialized beds in shelters for homeless individuals with chronic medical conditions who require more-intensive medical care, such as Christ House. There are also few services for homeless individuals with behavioral health needs and chronic medical conditions.

Finally, participants noted that many social and health interventions have failed in the past because of a lack of recognition of population literacy and trust issues. As one participant commented:

> Many projects have fallen dead due to inability to meet people where they're at. [For example,] they're surprised to learn that people can't read when trying to give them job training.

Participants also described how trust impacts the use of health and social services. Many hospitals and clinics have not established a trusting relationship with homeless and other vulnerable individuals. Such a relationship takes years to build. Interventions that fail to build this trust and promote sustainability by building community capacity will not succeed. Participants made the following comments relevant to this:

> [There is] distrust with the medical industry. It's not that just one hospital that needs to [address] it. They all need to attack it together, not separately.

> Will you come back next week? Communities are surprised when you come back. If the community does not accept or trust the project, you don't have a project.

5.11 Data Needs

We also asked participants about what data that they thought would be most helpful to included in D.C. Health Matters. In this section, we highlight the data needs they discussed.

Ward-Level Data
Participants felt that ward-level data, as well as hospital and ED data about chronic disease patterns, substance abuse, and mental health prevalence, would be helpful. In addition, information about utilization across demographics, such as race, is needed.

Community-Based Resources
Many participants felt that, in addition to data about health needs by ward, they would like to have access to a pathway that links such needs with the resources available to address these needs. As these resources can evolve rapidly, dedicated funding is needed to ensure that they are kept up to date.

Social Determinant Data
Many participants felt it would be useful to see data that linked health to social determinants. Suggestions included resources showing distance by ward to the nearest parks and bike lanes and mapping violent crime by location.

Data from Similar Jurisdictions
Having access to data from other similar cities would allow stakeholders to understand how D.C. residents fare compared to residents from other cities of similar size and demographic composition.

5.12 Summary Recommendations from Participants

We queried participants about recommendations of ways the DCHCC can improve health care and social services for District residents. This section presents some of these recommendations organized by topic.

Behavioral Health

Participants noted the need for additional behavioral health care services, particularly

- culturally appropriate primary and supportive services targeted toward persons for whom English is not a primary language
- services that promote independent living, such as housing, education, and training
- more skilled nursing facilities for persons with behavioral health needs and comorbid medical conditions to ease transition at the time of hospital discharge
- more housing options for the homeless with behavioral health needs
- greater provider awareness of and focus on associated comorbid medical conditions, such as HIV and viral hepatitis.

Obesity and Nutrition

Participants noted the need to inform residents through marketing approaches such as

- education about healthy eating options (such as healthy fruits and vegetables available in corner stores)
- education about existing community-based resources that promote fitness (such as Capital Bikeshare, parks, bike lanes)
- incorporating incentives to promote healthy behaviors, such as payment to parents to develop safe "walking school buses" (in which parents walk groups of children to school instead of using the bus), grocery store tours, cooking and exercise classes, and walking clubs.

Preventive Health

Participants thought that preventive health could be improved through the development of

- partnerships that link hospitals with social service organizations to promote healthy behavior (one example cited was hospitals allowing social organizations to offer exercise and fitness training directly on hospital grounds)
- programs that encourage the entire family to engage in healthy lifestyles, such as healthy shopping and family-targeted education initiatives, rather than addressing one age segment of the population.

Specialty Services

Participants suggested partnerships and incentives to promote the placement of providers in the community to supply needed specialty services. Examples included the use of loan repayment programs to motivate providers to work in community-based organizations, as well as the placement of medical physicians in training programs in neighborhood clinics and at non-profit social service sites.

Eldercare and End-of-Life Care

Participants noted the need for

- improved case management that supports the coordination of services for families who care for elderly relatives
- education about advanced directives.

Disability Services

Participants cited the need for more services for persons with disabilities, including

- programs that support persons with disabilities across the life continuum from infancy to adulthood
- improved case management services
- additional education for the medical community about the specific needs of persons with disabilities.

Information Technology

Participants noted the need for infrastructure to support the linkage of medical records across sites, such as programs like the DC RHIO.

Case Management and Care Coordination

Participants made a number of suggestions for improving case management, including

- expanded case management to link residents with medical services across hospitals, as well as with medical homes in the community
- the development of up-to-date lists of case management contacts at different facilities and the resources available in the community
- the use of lay patient navigators, such as those used in the cancer navigation model, to help link residents to appropriate community resources
- case management aimed at linking children to services as they transition into adulthood.

Social Determinants of Health

Participants also suggested a number of ways to address the social determinants of health, including

- improving awareness among the medical community of social determinants that impact health
- incorporating direct community exposure into provider training (e.g., through community-based medical school and residency rotations)
- expanding cultural competency training
- developing partnerships between hospitals and clinics and community-based organizations to help providers gain exposure to diverse populations
- developing partnerships between health care organizations and social organizations, such as faith-based establishments

- increasing hospital and FQHC presence in the community to educate patients about these resources, including the services available at particular sites
- educating the community about existing neighborhood resources using a streamlined, "one-stop shop" approach (e.g., health kiosks, resource lists including pertinent health and social service agency phone numbers made available at the time of discharge from a hospital)
- investing in housing and social service support for the homeless to reduce their use of hospital EDs when they lack food or shelter
- incorporating novel approaches targeted toward persons at varying literacy levels into health and social service interventions
- forming health and social partnerships that build social capital within the community rather than sending people from outside of the community to perform a service.

5.13 Summary

In general, our focus group findings largely paralleled the findings from our analysis of administrative data. There is a particular need for specialty services, including pain management services, which may explain the increase in pain-related visits to District EDs in recent years. The need for oncology services has been pointed out in prior RAND reports (Price et al., 2012). Services for certain populations, including residents in Wards 7 and 8, homeless individuals, persons with behavioral health needs, and immigrant and non–English-speaking residents are particularly in need. Participants also noted the need for more partnerships between social services agencies and hospitals and clinics to address the needs of many residents of the city.

CHAPTER SIX

Conclusions

In this section, we highlight our key findings in priority areas and identify gaps in knowledge. We determined priority areas using a combination of quantitative (administrative, survey) and qualitative (focus group) data analysis, as well as considering broader national health priority areas, paying particular attention to issues that have persisted over the last decade or experienced a recent increase or spike in the District. For example, we reviewed prior health needs assessments conducted in the District, exploring the trends in specific conditions or diagnoses. If those conditions persisted or assumed a new trend, we categorized them in the priority list. We then examined this list further, considering those issues that varied by at least one characteristic—age, ward, gender. We also examined areas in which need was high yet access to timely preventive care was poor, with particular disparities by age, race, and/or geographic area. While our choice of priority areas does not imply that other health areas do not require attention or investment (e.g., oral health), our analysis highlights that these are the top areas requiring primary intervention and the areas that have, in some cases, received less emphasis in prior health needs assessments.

6.1 Key Findings

The bulleted list below highlights key findings about health outcomes and access to health care among District residents. These findings should be of interest to all District hospitals and community health centers (see Appendix C).

The first priority area encompasses broader access-to-care issues, which underlie all other health conditions. The remaining five priority areas are organized by health condition.

Access to Care

Despite a high insurance rate in the District, there were several issues of access worthy of note.

- *District Versus the Overall United States.* The use of preventive health services was better in the District than it was nationally, with higher percentages of adults reporting a routine health care visit in the prior year and reporting a regular provider.
- *Age Differences.* More 18–39 and 40–64-year-olds missed care due to cost compared to those 65 years and older.
- *Race Differences.* Black residents reported more days of impairment than whites due to both mental health and physical health issues. Black residents also reported poorer health,

lower rates of flu and pneumococcal vaccination, and more missed care in the past 12 months due to cost than white residents.

- *Ward Differences.* There is significant variability in access to health care by ward, with Ward 1 having the highest percentage of individuals who report no routine medical visit in the prior year and Ward 5 having the highest percentage of individuals without a regular provider. Ward 8 has the highest percentage of persons who report difficulty in seeing a provider in the prior year due to cost.
- *Hospital Trends.* As a percentage of overall discharges, Children's National Medical Center experiences the most ACS inpatient discharges, followed by United Medical Center and Howard University Hospital. For Children's, this is driven by asthma and bacterial infections.
- *Stakeholder Perspectives.* In addition to the issues above, community stakeholders note concerns about the lack of behavioral health services, as well as the lack of specialists, particularly in the areas of oncology and pain management in Wards 7 and 8. Case management issues impede access to health and related social services. Hospitals and clinics do not offer many colocated services, and there is limited linkage across hospital sites. A lack of access to preventive care rather than treatment services alone was cited as a problem, inclusive of a lack of coordination between health and social services.

Health Conditions

Asthma

While other areas of health have experienced some improvements, this condition is the cause of many avoidable hospitalizations and ED visits.

- *District Versus the Overall United States.* Rates of asthma are higher in the District than they are nationally, both for adults and youth.
- *Age Differences.* Asthma rates are slightly higher among those 40–64 years old, followed by those 18–39 years old. Reports of asthma diagnoses increased between 2005 and 2011 for high school students, though it is unclear whether this was due to an increase in the condition or to improved detection.
- *Race Differences.* Black residents (both adults and youths) report higher levels of current asthma compared to white residents.
- *Ward Differences.* More individuals in Wards 5 and 7 report current asthma, and the lowest rates are in Wards 1 and 3.
- *Hospital Trends.* ACS inpatient discharges spiked after 2008 among those 0–17 years old and rates continue to be high for ACS ED discharges among this age group, primarily driven by asthma. ACS rates are highest among 0–17-year-old residents in Wards 7 and 8, though among 40–64-year-olds the rates are second highest in Wards 7 and 8. Children's National Medical Center experiences the bulk of these discharges.
- *Stakeholder Perspectives.* While asthma was not explicitly cited in the focus groups as a top priority issue, it did emerge in discussions regarding access to specialty care and difficulties in care coordination.

Obesity

Rates of obesity and overweight remain high in the District, but these rates cannot be explained solely by lack of physical activity.

- *District Versus the Overall United States.* Less District residents reported being overweight or obese than U.S. residents overall, and they were more likely to have engaged in exercise in the past 30 days.
- *Age Differences.* Rates of overweight and obesity were highest among those 40 years and older, and self-reported rates of getting enough exercise were lower among older adults than youth. More youth in the District did not exercise enough in the past week compared to youth nationally. Also, rates of self-reported obesity and overweight were higher among District youth, though gender differences were not significant.
- *Race Differences.* Black residents reported being overweight or obese more often than did white residents, and they were less likely to report vigorous exercise in the past month.
- *Ward Differences.* Obesity is more prevalent in Wards 7 and 8, while general overweight is more prevalent in Wards 4 and 5. Those in Wards 7 and 8 were the most infrequent reporters of exercise in the past 30 days, while those in Ward 3 were the most frequent.
- *Hospital Trends.* Obesity is not traditionally cited as the primary condition for inpatient or ED discharges. However, we know that heart disease and gastrointestinal issues, which are top conditions for discharges (see Appendix A), can be precipitated by weight issues.
- *Stakeholder Perspectives.* There is a shortage of family-targeted interventions that address obesity and promote healthy eating.

Sexual Health

In general, sexual health issues (beyond HIV testing rates and reductions in teen pregnancy) have remained a significant challenge in the District.

- *District Versus the Overall United States.* D.C. continues to report high STI rates relative to the U.S. population in chlamydia, syphilis, and gonorrhea. Hepatitis B and C are also of particular concern for the District and are commonly present together as coinfections or as coinfections in persons with HIV.
- *Age Differences.* STI rates among youth have increased over the last decade. Of all cases of chlamydia and gonorrhea reported in the District from 2006 through 2010, a significant proportion occurred among youth.
- *Ward Differences.* By ward over the five-year period from 2006 to 2010, rates of aggregate chlamydia and gonorrhea cases were highest in Wards 7 and 8 and lowest in Ward 3. Rates of primary and secondary syphilis cases were highest in Wards 1 and 2 and lowest in Ward 3 over that same period.
- *Hospital Trends.* In general, sexual health issues are not drivers of inpatient and ED discharges, though hepatitis and HIV are indicated as secondary reasons in some cases. In the related area of reproductive health, pregnancy complications are the top reason for inpatient discharges at Sibley Memorial Hospital.
- *Stakeholder Perspectives.* Individuals in focus groups noted the need for more resources devoted to educating residents about coinfections that occur with HIV, such as Hepatitis

B and C. Sexual health has also been discussed in prior stakeholder feedback sessions (see Chandra et al., 2009; Lurie et al., 2008).

Mental Health and Substance Use

These issues continue to be a concern to District stakeholders, with a particular focus on heavy drinking among young adults and poor access to behavioral health services.

- *District Versus the Overall United States.* Smoking is less common in the District compared to the overall United States. However, binge drinking and heavy drinking are more common.
- *Age Differences.* Smoking is most common among those aged 40–64 years, though heavy drinking and binge drinking is more common among those aged 18–39 years. The rate of marijuana use increased among high school youth from 2003 to 2011. The rate of feeling sad or hopeless has stayed fairly constant within 3 percentage points of the 2011 rate of 25 percent in the District. Rates of intimate partner violence and engagement in physical violence remain high among high school youth.
- *Race Differences.* Rates of depressive disorders are lower in the District than nationwide, with blacks reporting lower rates than whites.
- *Ward Differences.* Alcohol-related ED discharges are increasing among those 40–64 years old. For these discharges, the sharpest increase is among 18–39-year-olds living in Ward 1 and 40–64-years-olds in Wards 1 and 5.
- *Hospital Trends.* Generally, there are no major differences in mental health and substance use issues by hospital. However, United Medical Center reports a high rate of inpatient discharges due to schizophrenia, and Howard University Hospital reports the most discharges among 18–64-year-olds related to alcohol.
- *Stakeholder Perspectives.* Behavioral health services are limited for persons with Medicaid, as well as for persons for whom English is not their primary language. Treatment options for comorbid medical conditions associated with behavioral health issues are also limited.

Stress-Related Diagnoses

A key trend in ED discharges over the past few years has been in the area of "stress-related discharges," namely headaches, migraines, and back pain. Data for these conditions are not easily comparable with national data or by race, so those comparisons are not listed.

- *Age Differences.* The rate of back-pain ED discharges has sharply increased, especially among those 40–64 years old. Headache and migraine issues are also highest among those 40–64 years old, followed by those 65 and older and those 18–39 years old.
- *Ward Differences.* This increase in back pain ED discharges, headache, and migraine issues appears to be greatest among those 40–64 years old in Wards 5, 6, and 7 and less common in Wards 2 and 3. Similarly, headache and migraine discharges have increased (since 2009) among those 40–64 years old, particularly in Wards 5 and 7.
- *Hospital Trends.* George Washington University Hospital, Washington Hospital Center, Providence Hospital, and Howard University Hospital report the most back-pain ED discharges. The same hospital patterns persist for migraines as well.

- *Stakeholder Perspectives.* Access to pain management specialty care is limited, particularly in Wards 7 and 8.

6.2 Gaps in Knowledge and Limitations

In this section, we highlight a few gaps in knowledge, as well as some limitations. Please note that, due to limited resources and scope, we did not delve into these issues fully, but future analyses could explore these topics further. We divide this discussion into two sections covering broad data issues and specific analyses by condition.

Broad Data Issues
Access to Data Continues to Be a Concern
While we were able to obtain data from the D.C. Hospital Association, these data are not publicly available without special request, thus limiting the ability of various stakeholders to review trends over time. In addition, we were unable to easily access other ED data (e.g., United Medical Center), which would have rounded out our analyses, particularly regarding trends in pediatric conditions. Additional access to community health center data would aid health care planners, but to date, those data are not readily accessible.

Hospital and ED Data Have Limitations
While analyses of hospital discharge data provide a good snapshot of the use of hospital services, it does not provide a complete picture of health need in a community because the data only capture service seeking where there is an actual admission. Further, we used the condition classification codes for primary diagnoses only, although we know there are secondary and tertiary conditions that may drive hospital or ED use.

Primary Care Analyses Would Benefit from Better Information on Provider Supply
This report did not conduct a broader analysis of primary care supply, which has implications for the ability to access and use timely preventive care (as shown by ACS rates). Supply data are limited by the quality of physician and other health care provider information, particularly information on the amount of time in practice in the District specifically.

Health-Need Data Captured by BRFSS And YRBS Are Limited by the Lack of Subcity Information
While BRFSS data have been analyzed by ward, YRBS data are not available at the ward level, which precludes more nuanced analyses of health need among youth. Further, while there are strong efforts to analyze these data quickly, analyses are somewhat lagged due to time delays in cleaning, assessing, and disseminating the data. More timely analyses of this information would improve local health planning.

Condition-Specific Analyses
It Is Unclear What Contributes to Declines in Discharges Due to Coronary Atherosclerosis
As we noted in this analysis, there has been a sharp decline in discharges due to this heart condition. We cannot yet determine if this is due to improved and timely care; the use of medica-

tions; more extensive management of these patients in EDs, thus avoiding admission; and/or a shift of these patients to outpatient or specialty care settings.

More Information Needs to Be Captured on What Is Contributing to High Rates of Heavy and Binge Drinking and Alcohol-Related ED Visits

Based on further analyses, it appears that college students and other adults are contributing to sharp increases in these rates. Given that the college student population has not changed markedly, these increases may also be due to demographic transitions and the increase in the percentage of the population below 39 years old. More research is needed.

It Is Necessary to Understand Care Coordination and Health and Social Service Linkage Issues in Further Detail

The issue of care coordination was a robust theme in all focus groups. Further investigation would be useful to understand how to strengthen care coordination across hospitals, identify models that are most effective, and determine how to streamline and colocate services in high-need areas.

There Are Limited Data on Child Oral Health

Most of the data in this report are a few years old, and updates to the 2011 National Survey of Children's Health data (as an example) are not yet available. Determining a way to more regularly gather data on oral health, and specifically child oral health, is critical.

6.3 Summary

Overall, many of the same issues that were present in prior CHNAs, including asthma, obesity, mental health, and sexual health issues, have been illustrated in this most recent version. Despite high insurance rates in the District, services (both prevention and specialty) are not evenly distributed by ward, creating significant access challenges. Further, care coordination issues across health and social services are a significant concern that has not received as much attention.

Each priority condition or topic suggests particular pathways. For access to care, District attention to narrowing the gap in racial/ethnic disparities in access to preventive care still merits intervention. Further, there are potentially a few solutions in certain areas of preventive care access that may require a comparatively modest effort, such as improving the pneumococcal vaccine rates among older residents. In addition, better integration of health and social services may help facilitate timely use of preventive health services, creating new access points (i.e., via social services) for individuals to obtain primary care. With regard to asthma, ACS rates are still high, suggesting that improvements in care coordination may facilitate more timely asthma management, particularly among those 0–17 years old. For obesity, there may be two targets of intervention. First, those who are overweight may benefit from intense engagement to ensure they do not move to "obese" status. Plus, the lack of access to and involvement in more regular exercise is a problem, specifically among adults 40 years and older. Determining ways to disseminate exercise opportunities to these age groups should be a priority. In the area of sexual health, STI rates remain alarmingly high, particularly the rates of chlamydia and gonorrhea among District youth. More education about the co-occurrence of HIV and hepatitis B and C, as well as the education of youth about the long-term sequelae of gonorrhea and chlamydia among District youth are needed. For mental health and substance use, more attention may be needed in the area of alcohol-related discharges among 18–39-year-olds, given the recent spike in those discharges. In addition, access to behavioral health services remains a high stakeholder priority, particularly for vulnerable populations, including the homeless and non–English-speaking residents. Stress-related discharges, defined by headaches, migraines, and backaches, may also be a trend worthy of note. In many instances, these conditions are the somatic precursors for more significant mental or behavioral health issues.

In addition to these intervention pathways by priority health condition, we identified emerging issues that require further investigation. First, the sharp increase in asthma-related discharges after years of decline merits analysis. In addition, further study should be done to evaluate the decline in coronary atherosclerosis discharges. Also, the new spike in stress-related diagnoses (headaches and back pain) and associated alcohol-related issues warrant additional analysis and intervention. This may be related to a host of factors, including economic downturn and demographic transitions in the District.

Top 20 Primary Conditions for Inpatient and ED Discharges (2007–2011 rankings)

Table A.1
Inpatient Discharges

Primary Condition (using Condition Classification System)	Rank (based on total discharges)				
	2007	2008	2009	2010	2011
[07.02] Diseases of the heart	1	1	1	1	1
[16.10] Complications	2	2	2	2	2
[11.03] Complications mainly related to pregnancy	3	3	3	3	3
[10.01] Diseases of the urinary system	8	7	7	6	4
[07.03] Cerebrovascular disease	5	5	4	4	5
[11.04] Indications for care in pregnancy; labor; and delivery	6	6	5.5	5	6
[05.08] Mood disorders	9	10	8	9	7
[09.06] Lower gastrointestinal disorders	11	12	11	11	8
[11.06] Other complications of birth; puerperium affecting management of mother	7	8	9	8	9
[16.02] Fractures	10	9	10	10	10
[08.01] Respiratory infections	15	11	12	13	11
[03.03] Diabetes mellitus with complications	13	15	14	12	12
[05.10] Schizophrenia and other psychotic disorders	17	13	15	15	13
[07.01] Hypertension	19	20	17	21	14
[17.01] Symptoms; signs; and ill-defined conditions	4	4	5.5	7	15

Table A.2
ED Discharges

Primary Condition (using Condition Classification System)	Rank (based on total discharges)				
	2007	2008	2009	2010	2011
[17.01] Symptoms; signs; and ill-defined conditions	1	1	1	1	1
[08.01] Respiratory infections	2	2	2	2	2
[16.08] Superficial injury; contusion	5	6	7	4	3
[16.07] Sprains and strains	4	3	4	3	4
[16.06] Open wounds	3	4	6	6	5
[07.02] Diseases of the heart	6	5	3	5	6
[06.08] Ear conditions	13	10	9	9	7
[13.03] Spondylosis; intervertebral disc disorders; other back problems	12	11	10	7	8
[10.01] Diseases of the urinary system	8	8	8	8	9
[16.12] Other injuries and conditions due to external causes	7	7	5	11	10
[17.02] Factors influencing health care	9	9	11	10	11
[13.08] Other connective tissue disease	10	12	12	12	12
[13.02] Non-traumatic joint disorders	16	16	18	13	13
[06.05] Headache; including migraine	15	15	16	15	14
[16.02] Fractures	17	17	19	18	15

Health and Social Determinants Focus Group Protocols

Health Focus Group Protocol

Overview of Health Care Needs in the City

We realize that each of you represent unique organizations with specific targeted populations. We would first like for you to start by thinking broadly and to think about priority health needs in the city as a whole. Let's start by discussing your opinions of priority health and health care issues in general.

1. From your perspective, what are priority HEALTH issues in this city? Where do you see the greatest improvement in addressing these issues (type of issue, age group, location)? Where is more work needed?
2. What are priority HEALTH SERVICE needs in the city?
3. Thinking about these priority HEALTH SERVICE needs, which particular ones has the health care community in the city addressed particularly well?
   a. What targeted populations in particular have benefitted? (probe age groups, chronic disease subsets, gender)
   b. What targeted locations of the city have most benefitted?

4. Thinking about these priority HEALTH SERVICE needs, which particular ones need more attention and action from the city's health care community?
   a. What targeted populations need more attention? (probe age groups, chronic disease subsets, gender)
   b. What targeted locations of the city need more attention?

Stakeholder Work

Now we would like to talk about your work in providing health care services, specifically, in the District to the particular population you serve through your organization.

1. What are the greatest health and health service needs of the population you serve?
   a. What additional health care services are needed to address these health issues?
   b. Can you give some examples of types of programs that would help?

2. What barriers do you find in delivering services to your population to address these health care needs? (probe social support services, networking, funding)

Recommendations for DCHCC

Now, we would like to get your recommendations on what DCHCC can do to improve care for the city? Please try to think as concretely as possible.

1. Thinking about the DCHCC's member hospitals and FQHCs, what can it do to help improve health service delivery for the population you serve?
2. What can DCHCC do to help improve general social service delivery for the population you serve?

Prioritization of Recommendations

1. If you had to prioritize these recommendations, what are your top 3 or 5? Ask participants to rank on their own sheet of paper first, then lead discussion of why they chose these 3 or 5.
2. What do you think would have the most impact on health in the city? Why?
3. What do you think would have the greatest impact on the population you serve?

Partnership

1. In what ways can your organization partner with DCHCC members to improve social service and health needs in the city, please think of some concrete suggestions?
2. What are some barriers to this partnership?
3. What can the DCHCC do to facilitate this partnership?

Data Needs
[If time permits...]

Now, we would like you to think about your data needs as a provider of health care services in the city.

1. What kind of data do you find you need most often in your work?
    a. For what purposes do you need this data?
    b. Where do you usually find your data?
    c. What data do you find is most accessible?
    d. What data do you need that you often have difficulty finding?

[write on board or flip chart so group can see suggestions]

Social Determinants Focus Group Protocol

Overview of Social Service Needs in the City

We realize that each of you represent unique organizations with specific targeted populations. We would first like for you to start by thinking broadly and to think about priority social service needs in the city as a whole and how these needs impact the health of the city's residents. Let's start by discussing your opinions of priority social needs of the city in general.

1. From your perspective, what are priority social service needs in the city as a whole?
   a. How do these social service needs impact the health of the city's residents?
2. Thinking about these priority SOCIAL SERVICE needs, which particular ones has the city addressed particularly well?
   a. What targeted populations in particular have benefitted?
   b. What targeted locations of the city have most benefitted?
3. Thinking about these priority SOCIAL SERVICE needs, which particular ones need more attention and action from the city?
   a. What targeted populations need more attention? (probe age groups, chronic disease subsets)
   b. What targeted locations of the city need more attention?

Stakeholder Work

Now we would like to talk about your work in providing social services in the District to the particular population you serve through your organization.

1. What are the greatest social service needs of the specific population you serve?
2. Now let's think about how these social service needs impact the health of the population you serve. What general social factors are not being addressed which would improve the health of your population?
3. What types of services would that entail?
4. What barriers do you find in delivering services to your population to address these social service needs? [probe social support services, networking, funding]

Recommendations for DCHCC

Now, we would like to get your recommendations on what DCHCC can do to improve care for the city? Please try to think as concretely as possible.

1. Thinking about the DCHCC's member hospitals and FQHCs, what can it do to help address the social factors that affect health of the population you serve?
2. What can DCHCC with other organizations to address the social factors that relate to health outcomes among the population you serve?

Prioritization of Recommendations

1. If you had to prioritize these recommendations, what are your top 3 or 5? [Ask participants to rank on their own sheet of paper first, then lead discussion of why they chose these 3 or 5 on board or flip chart to come up with a consensus.]
2. What do you think would have the most impact on health in the city as a whole? Why?
3. What do you think would have the greatest impact on the population you serve?

Partnership

1. In what ways can your organization partner with DCHCC members to improve social service and health needs in the city? (please think of some concrete suggestions)
2. What are some barriers to this partnership?
3. What can the DCHCC do to facilitate this partnership?

Data Needs
[If time permits…]

Now, we would like you to think about your data needs as a provider of social services in the city.

1. What kind of data do you find you need most often in your work?
   a. For what purposes do you need this data?
   b. Where do you usually find your data?
   c. What data do you find is most accessible?
   d. What data do you need that you often have difficulty finding?

[write on board or flip chart so group can see suggestion]

District of Columbia Hospitals and Community Health Centers

Hospital and community health centers in D.C. are committed to addressing community health needs. A list of D.C. hospitals is listed below and community health centers are noted on the D.C. Primary Care Association website (http://www.dcpca.org/health-centers/):

- Children's National Medical Center
- George Washington University Hospital
- Georgetown University Hospital
- Hospital for Sick Children
- Howard University Hospital
- National Rehabilitation Hospital
- Providence Hospital
- Psychiatric Institute of Washington
- Sibley Memorial Hospital
- Specialty Hospital of Washington—Capitol Hill
- Specialty Hospital of Washington—Hadley
- St. Elizabeth's Hospital
- United Medical Center (formerly Greater Southeast Community Hospital)
- Washington Hospital Center.

References

Austin, S. Bryn, S. J. Melly, B. N. Sanchez, et al., "Clustering of Fast-Food Restaurants Around Schools: A Novel Application of Spatial Statistics to the Study of Food Environment," *American Journal of Public Health*, Vol. 95, No. 9, September 2005, pp. 1575–1581.

BRFSS—*See* District of Columbia Department of Health, June 2012.

CDC WONDER, "Bridged Race Population Estimates: United States, States, and Country for the Years 1990–2011," October 26, 2012. As of February 23, 2013:
http://wonder.cdc.gov/wonder/help/bridged-race.html

Centers for Medicare and Medicaid Services, *Annual EPSDT Participation Report—District of Columbia FY: 2010*, Baltimore, Md.: U.S. Department of Health and Human Services, 2011.

Chandra, A., C. R. Gresenz, J. Blanchard, A. Cuellar, T. Ruder, et al., *Health and Health Care Among District of Columbia Youth*, Santa Monica, Calif.: RAND Corporation, TR-751-CNMC, 2009.

Cohen, Deborah A., Thomas L. McKenzie, Amber Sehgal, Stephanie Williamson, Daniela Golinelli, and Nicole Lurie, "Contribution of Public Parks to Physical Activity," *American Journal of Public Health*, Vol. 97, No. 3, March 2007, pp. 509–514.

Data Resource Center for Child and Adolescent Health, National Survey of Children's Health, 2012. As of December 10, 2012:
http://www.childhealthdata.org/learn/NSCH

De Bordeau Huij, I., J. F. Sallis, B. Saelens, "Environmental Correlates of Physical Activity in a Sample of Belgian Adults," *American Journal of Health Promotion*, Vol. 18, No. 1, September/October 2003, pp. 83–92.

District of Columbia Department of Health, *HIV/AIDS, Hepatitis, STD, and TB Epidemiology in the District of Columbia*, 2011.

District of Columbia Department of Health, *BRFSS 2010 Annual Health Report*, June 2012. As of December 12, 2012:
http://doh.dc.gov/sites/default/files/dc/sites/doh/publication/attachments/BRFSS_Annual_Report_2010.pdf

District of Columbia Department of Health, Data Management and Analysis Division, Center for Policy, Planning, and Evaluation, *2010 Infant Mortality Rate for the District of Columbia*, April 26, 2012.

District of Columbia Metropolitan Police Department, "District Crime at a Glance," January 24, 2013. As of January 24, 2013:
http://mpdc.dc.gov/page/district-crime-data-glance

Federal Bureau of Investigation, *Uniform Crime Reports*, undated. As of January 10, 2013:
http://www.fbi.gov/about-us/cjis/ucr/ucr

Freisthler, B., L. Ring, P. J. Gruenwald, et al., "An Ecological Assessment of the Population and Environmental Correlates of Childhood Accident, Assault and Child Abuse Injuries," *Alcoholism: Clinical and Experimental Research*, Vol. 32, No. 11, 2008, pp. 1969–1975.

Giles-Corti, B., and R. J. Donovan, The Relative Influence of Individual, Social Environmental, and Physical Environmental Correlates of Walking, *American Journal of Public Health*, Vol. 93, No. 9, September 2003, pp. 1152–1158.

Gresenz, Carole Roan, Janice C. Blanchard, Justin W. Timbie, et al., *Behavioral Health in the District of Columbia: Assessing Need and Evaluating the Public System of Care*, Santa Monica, Calif.: RAND Corporation, TR-914-DCDMH, 2010.

Gruenewald, P. J., and L. Remer, "Changes in Outlet Densities Affect Violence Rates," *Alcoholism: Clinical and Experimental Research*, Vol. 30, No. 7, July 2006, pp. 1184–1193.

Kaiser Family Foundation, State Health Facts, "District of Columbia: Facts At-a-Glance," undated. As of February 4, 2013:
http://www.statehealthfacts.org/profileglance.jsp?rgn=10.

Lurie, N., C. R. Gresenz, J. Blanchard, T. Ruder, A. Chandra, et al., *Assessing Health and Health Care in the District of Columbia*, Santa Monica, Calif.: RAND Corporation, WR-534, 2008. As of May 1, 2013:
http://www.rand.org/pubs/working_papers/WR534.html

Martin, J. A., B. E. Hamilton, S. J. Ventura, M. K. Osterman, E. C. Wilson, and T. J. Matthews, "Births: Final Data for 2010," *National Vital Statistics Reports*, Vol. 61, No. 1, August 28, 2012. As of December 15, 2012:
http://www.cdc.gov/nchs/data/nvsr/nvsr61/nvsr61_01.pdf#table01

McGee, Daniel L., Youlian Liao, Guichan Cao, and Richard S. Cooper, "Self-Reported Health Status and Mortality in a Multiethnic U.S. Cohort," *American Journal of Epidemiology*, Vol. 149, No. 1, 1999, pp. 41–46.

National Cancer Institute, *State Cancer Profiles*, undated. As of January 16, 2012:
http://statecancerprofiles.cancer.gov/cgi-bin/quickprofiles/profile.pl?11&515

Price, Rebecca Anhang, Janice C. Blanchard, Racine Harris, Teague Ruder, and Carole Roan Gresenz, *Monitoring Cancer Outcomes Across the Continuum: Data Synthesis and Analysis for the District of Columbia*, Santa Monica, Calif.: RAND Corporation, TR-1296-DCCC, 2012. As of April 14, 2013:
http://www.rand.org/pubs/technical_reports/TR1296

Roemmich, J. N., L. H. Epstein, S. Raja, et al., "Association of Access to Parks and Recreational Facilities with the Physical Activity of Young Children," *Preventive Medicine*, Vol. 43, No. 6, December 2006, pp. 437–441.

Sallis, J. F., and N. Owen, "Ecological Models," in Karen Ganz, Frances Lewis, and Barbara Rimer, eds., *Health Behavior and Health Education: Theory, Research, and Practice*, New York: Jossey-Bass, 1990.

SAMHSA, "2010–2011 National Survey on Drug Use and Health Model-Based Estimates," undated. As of February 4, 2013:
http://www.samhsa.gov/data/NSDUH/2k11State/NSDUHsaeTables2011.pdf

U.S. Census Bureau, American Community Survey 2006–2010, 2011. As of May 1, 2013:
http://www.census.gov/acs/www/

U.S. Census Bureau, Decennial Census, 2000.

U.S. Department of Health and Human Services, Health Resources and Services Administration, "Shortage Designation: Health Professional Shortage Areas & Medically Underserved Areas/Populations," 2012. As of December 10, 2012:
http://bhpr.hrsa.gov/shortage/